.

# Cystatin C and Kidney Stone Disease - Updating Evidence-Based Data and Future Perspectives

*Edited by Giovanni Palleschi
and Valeria Rossi*

Published in London, United Kingdom

Cystatin C and Kidney Stone Disease - Updating Evidence-Based Data and Future Perspectives
http://dx.doi.org/10.5772/intechopen.1003482
Edited by Giovanni Palleschi and Valeria Rossi

Contributors

Alessandro Calarco, Chukwuka Azubuike, Elias David-Neto, Flávia S. Reis, Giovanni Palleschi, John Emenike Anieche, Manish Bhatia, Ngozi Eucheria Makata, Pietro Viscuso, Smita Kumbhar, Valeria Rossi

Notice

Statements and opinions expressed in the chapters are these of the individual contributors and not necessarily those of the editors or publisher. No responsibility is accepted for the accuracy of information contained in the published chapters. The publisher assumes no responsibility for any damage or injury to persons or property arising out of the use of any materials, instructions, methods or ideas contained in the book.

First published in London, United Kingdom, 2025 by IntechOpen
IntechOpen is the global imprint of INTECHOPEN LIMITED, registered in England and Wales, registration number: 11086078, 167-169 Great Portland Street, London, W1W 5PF, United Kingdom

For EU product safety concerns: IN TECH d.o.o., Prolaz Marije Krucifikse Kozulić 3, 51000 Rijeka, Croatia, info@intechopen.com or visit our website at intechopen.com.

British Library Cataloguing-in-Publication Data
A catalogue record for this book is available from the British Library

Cystatin C and Kidney Stone Disease - Updating Evidence-Based Data and Future Perspectives
Edited by Giovanni Palleschi and Valeria Rossi
p. cm.
Print ISBN 978-0-85466-290-6
Online ISBN 978-0-85466-289-0
eBook (PDF) ISBN 978-0-85466-291-3

If disposing of this product, please recycle the paper responsibly.

# Meet the editors

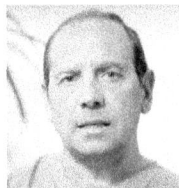

Giovanni Palleschi (MD, Ph.D.) graduated in Medicine in 1997 and specialized in Urology in 2002, both at Sapienza University of Rome, where he gained a grant for research on voiding disorders in patients with Multiple Sclerosis (2002) and completed a physician doctorate in human anatomy, plastic surgery and dermatology in 2011. In his career, he attended a Master's in Laparoscopic Surgery in Strasbourg (IRCAD), an International Master's in Laparoscopy (Sapienza University of Rome and Carol Davila University of Bucharest), and a Master's in Kidney Transplant at Tor Vergata University of Rome. He has been a member of the Scientific Committees for the Italian Society of Urodynamics, the European Association of Urology, and the Italian Society of Urology. He has served as a co-investigator in numerous clinical trials and as a Scientific Consultant for various pharmaceutical companies. He has published numerous articles on PubMed and is an author and co-author of various scientific books. He won 6 Scientific Awards, and participated in Academic Activities (teaching) for the Sapienza University of Rome. At present, he works in Italy for the Nefrocenter Group.

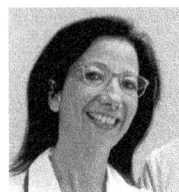

Valeria Rossi, MD, graduated in Medicine in 2000 from Sapienza University of Rome. She then specialized in Nephrology at Tor Vergata University of Rome in 2005. In her career, she has gained extensive experience as Chief of Nephrology and Dialysis Units since 2009, including expertise in the surgical management of vascular accesses for patients undergoing hemodialysis. She has published numerous manuscripts on chronic kidney disease, with a focus on diabetic nephropathy and techniques for hemodialysis. She is frequently invited to speak at various national nephrology congresses and has participated as an author, co-author, and editor in several publications and scientific books. Currently, she serves as the Chief of the Hemodialysis Unit at Frascati (Rome) for the Nefrocenter Group.

# Contents

# Preface

Renal failure has a significant epidemiological and socioeconomic impact in all countries, and its prevalence is increasing over the years. This is the consequence of the strong incidence of comorbidities that represent potential causes of kidney failure, particularly high blood pressure, dyslipidemia, diabetes, and obesity. In addition, the growing incidence of neoplastic conditions that need the administration of chemotherapies that have nephrotoxicity, and some wrong diet habits (hyperproteic, hypercaloric), have recently contributed to kidney damage in the general population. Acute and chronic kidney disease are both associated with an increased risk of death, therefore requiring attention by public healthcare in terms of primary prevention programs. Diagnostic and therapeutic management of renal failure imposes a severe economic burden on societies, and the need for recurrent laboratory exams, instrumental diagnostic procedures (especially ultrasound), and administration of expensive drugs are all responsible for significant economic loss every year for the sanitary systems. However, the most important cost-related rate of kidney failure is represented by replacement therapies (dialysis) and kidney transplant. Considering all this data and the expected growth of population in the coming decades, kidney failure could become, by 2040, the fifth cause of death. This is one of the main reasons why a strong effort is being made in the fields of diagnosis and treatment of acute and chronic renal failure in all countries. Many resources have been collected in the last years to prompt research aiming to improve early diagnosis of kidney failure and its management, to reduce the risk of End Stage Renal Disease, that needs replacement therapies, that are not only associated to high costs but also to a significant reduction of both quality of life and life-expectancy. A better management of this condition, from early diagnosis to treatment, has been achieved using serum parameters and molecular markers. Cystatin C has been used for many years as a reliable marker of kidney function, as it is considered independent of factors such as patient sex and weight. Recent research has introduced new insights into the use of Cystatin C in the field of kidney disease, with the most important findings reported in this book. After an Introductory Chapter (Chapter 1) that resumes some historical data about Cystatin C and provides an overview of data from the literature on the argument, new significant insights about the use of Cystatin C in clinical practice are described in Chapter 2. In this chapter, the contribution of Cystatin C to monitoring acute and chronic conditions is reported, and recent data from basic research studies are provided, especially to explain how this molecular marker may aid in decision-making processes. Living in the modern era and dealing with Artificial Intelligence is described in Chapter 3, which discusses the possible contribution of Big Data and Artificial Intelligence Systems to investigate and use knowledge on Cystatin C for clinical purposes (from diagnostic goals to predictive role in pathological conditions).

A significant rate of patients with chronic kidney disease is represented by those suffering from kidney stones. The role that urolithiasis plays in determining chronic kidney failure is still underestimated. Patients often require recurrent surgical treatments to achieve a stone-free condition, and this increases the risk of cumulative kidney damage over time. However, significant innovations in the surgical treatment of urinary stones have significantly improved various aspects of the therapeutic approach, including better outcomes, shorter operative times, fewer procedures, and a lower risk of major complications. These topics are reported in Chapters 4 and 5, which describe new insights about the use of percutaneous nephrolithotomy and the management of nephrolithiasis. These contributions offer a significant update in the field of kidney disease, reporting data with practical applications in daily clinical practice. It is my pleasure to thank all the authors of this book's chapters for their support and valuable contributions, especially for their efforts in improving knowledge in the field of kidney disease.

**Giovanni Palleschi, MD, PhD, Urologist and Valeria Rossi, MD, Nephrologist**
Nefrocenter Group,
Frascati (Rome), Italy

Chapter 1

# Introductory Chapter: Cystatin C – Overview of Main Clinical and Research Issues

*Giovanni Palleschi and Valeria Rossi*

## 1. Introduction

The use of molecular markers for diagnostic and prognostic purposes has increased in recent years due to various factors. First of all, this is the result of a significant effort in base research that has produced innovative data about the involvement of these markers in the pathophysiologic mechanisms of various disorders; secondarily, there is strong evidence that the use of molecular biomarkers may contribute to reducing invasive examinations in the pre-clinical stage of pathological conditions, it helps to achieve earlier diagnosis of many disorders with consequent better therapeutic results [1]. Generally, molecular biomarkers (also known as "signature molecules") are represented by circulating proteins that can be identified by immunoenzymatic techniques [2]. Clinicians are prompting large research on biomarkers because these molecules can be the key to the biomanufacturing of therapeutic proteins. In the future, the use of nanotechnologies for treating pathologic conditions will surely increase, and the adoption of biomarkers for diagnosis, prognosis, and developing proteins with therapeutic properties could really represent a "new scenario" of molecular-target therapies [2]. In fact, various manuscripts already available from the literature report data regarding the use of biomarkers and disease-modifying therapies [3]. Among molecular markers of large use in clinical practice, cystatin C has shown in the last years a significant increase. Cystatin C is a 13,343-Dalton protein and it consists of 120 amino acid residues in a single polypeptide chain. It is a non-glycosylated basic protein having an isoelectric point of pH 9.3, with a structure made by a short alpha helix and a long alpha helix lying on a large antiparallel, five-stranded beta-sheet [4]. This structure is quite similar to that of type 2 cystatins, and it contains two disulfide bonds. Cystatin C was first described in 1961 and its structure and aminoacidic sequence were reported by Grubb and Lofberg [4]. These researchers were those who found that the cystatin C levels were high in subjects with renal failure [5] and subsequent studies investigated and then proposed its use as a measure of glomerular filtration rate [6]. During the following years, a large number of clinical trials have been performed to assess the role of cystatin C as a biomarker of renal function, and of kidney acute and chronic disease. Nowadays, cystatin C is widely used in clinical nephrology and its measurement represents one of the most important diagnostic and prognostic factors of kidney disease. Since cystatin C is produced by all nucleated cells in the body, research on this biomarker has subsequently extended to other fields of medicine. Many investigations support the role of cystatin C as a potential marker of cardiovascular disease, ischemic stroke, endocrinological alterations (especially thyroid diseases), neurological degenerative disorders (Alzheimer's disease), diabetes mellitus, pulmonary and systemic infections (COVID-19 included), chronic obstructive pulmonary disease, oncologic conditions (risk of cancer progression and urological malignancies). Furthermore, some studies support the evidence of a correlation between cystatin C levels and mortality risk in the general population.

## 2. Cystatin C: Fields of application

The most important field of clinical application of cystatin C is the assessment of glomerular filtration rate. A large number of studies, systematic reviews, and meta-nalysis published in literature support this evidence, confirming the high diagnostic accuracy of this biomarker and its more sensitiveness for the estimation of glomeru-lar filtration rate when the cut-off value is set to 60 ml/min/1.73m$^2$ [7]. Recently, favorable data about the predictive role of cystatin C in glomerular filtration rate and patients receiving kidney transplants has been demonstrated [8]. The use of cystatin C has been shown to be highly predictive also of acute kidney injury in adults and in children [9]. Furthermore, the latest data strongly underline how important the use of cystatin C is, particularly in the early stages of kidney disease, prompting its measurement in individuals for whom the assessment of creatinine appears inad-equate [10]. Therefore, in nephrology at present time, there is the most important use of cystatin C either for clinical applications and for research purposes. The diffusion of knowledge about this biomarker has prompted research in other medical fields. Several studies have focused on the potential diagnostic and prognostic role of cys-tatin C in cardiovascular disorders. The results of specific metanalysis on this topic suggest that cystatin C may be considered as an independent predictor of cardio-vascular mortality in the general population: high levels of cystatin C are associated with an increased cardiovascular risk of death [11]. Regarding coronary disease, Jun Chen et al. described, after a meta-analysis, that higher levels of cystatin C in the blood are associated with a significantly higher risk of acute myocardial infarction. This study examined eight large investigations including 7394 patients and suggested that plasmatic levels of cystatin C could be stratified and become predictive of the success of revascularization procedures [12]. Among vascular diseases, ischemic stroke has been found to be in relationship with cystatin C. A recent study performed in 2019 by Yan Wang et al. reported the outcomes of a meta-analysis designed to assess if cystatin C levels might be predictive of ischemic stroke. The review of these studies, comprehensive of a total number of 3773 patients, revealed an association between cystatin C levels and ischemic stroke, specifically acute ischemic stroke and subclinical cerebral infarction, inducing the authors to conclude that this protein could be considered a predictor of both these clinical conditions [13]. This finding correlates well with the increased levels of cystatin C found in patients suffering from atherosclerosis, which represents one of the most important causes of ischemic stroke [14]. Systematic reviews have also demonstrated that cystatin C levels are higher in subjects suffering from type 2 diabetes mellitus with respect to healthy individuals [15], and the same for those affected by hyperthyroidism [16] and chronic obstruc-tive pulmonary disease [17]. These evidences support the concept that the protease system is stimulated and activated by various factors, either inflammatory or toxic (as an increase in blood levels of specific molecules). More recent investigations have provided evidence that cystatin C levels may significantly vary in some neurologic disorders. As already known, alterations of proteolytic mechanisms develop during aging process and have been discovered in some pathological conditions that involve the central nervous system. Therefore also the inhibition of cysteine protease can undergo significant changes in these conditions. In fact, many studies reveal important modifications of cystatin C concentrations in neural tissues of subjects affected by pathological conditions of the nervous system. This finding has been proven either in experimental models or in specimens obtained from patients suffering from neurodegenerative disorders, first of all, Alzheimer's disease [18]. When the proteolytic activity is high, tissue degeneration is accelerated, and pathophysiologic mechanisms of neural damage are exacerbated. Therefore, a favorable, protective effect of cystatin C against degenerative mechanisms involved in Alzheimer's disease has been proved [18]. In particular, cystatin C seems to play a protective role in preventing the aggregation of beta-amyloid, which is one of the most important histopathological finding in tissues of subjects affected by Alzheimer's disease [19]. In fact, various studies have shown that cystatin C levels in the blood may be predictive of the risk of cognitive impairment and dementia [20]. Some other studies have provided evidence that cystatin C levels increase during systemic conditions, such as obesity or infectious disorders (including the SARS-CoV-2 infective disease) [14, 21]. Among various physiologic and pathophysiologic mechanisms, cystatin C appears to be involved in the cancer progression of various human tumors, even if literature provides data that still appear controversial about this topic [22]. However, it has been shown that cystatin C can represent an indicator for the diagnosis of myeloma nephropathy, reflecting tumor burden and being associated with the prognosis of this condition [23]. In the oncologic field, there is also evidence that cystatin C might become a biomarker of urogenital neoplastic diseases. Some studies have investigated the expression of cystatin C in the serum and tissues in patients with renal cell carcinoma, the presence of cystatin C in the urine, tissues, and serum of those with prostatic cancer, in the serum of those with bladder cancers and other urogenital malignancies (urothelial carcinoma) [24]. These studies are not conclusive, but they give an enthusiastic perspective on the chance of using cystatin C as a predictive biomarker of urogenital tumors in the near future.

## 3. Conclusion

Data reported above clearly show that there is a significant effort made by clinicians and researchers to find out the role of cystatin C in the pathophysiologic mechanisms of numerous pathological clinical conditions. Despite the hard evidence that cystatin C is a strong biomarker of acute and chronic renal failure, thus making its use very common in nephrological clinical practice, this is not the same in other medical fields. This book will explore the most recent evidence provided by clinical and base research on cystatin C, aiming to provide the most complete update on this topic nowadays available in literature.

## Author details

Giovanni Palleschi* and Valeria Rossi
NEFROCENTER Hemodialysis Company, Frascati, Rome, Italy

*Address all correspondence to: giovanni.palleschi@santagostino.it

IntechOpen

# References

[1] Hong H, Goodsaid F, Shi L, Tong W. Molecular biomarkers: A US FDA effort. Biomarkers in Medicine. 2010;**4**(2): 215-225. DOI: 10.2217

[2] Desmurget C, Perilleux A, Souquet J, Borth N, Douet J. Molecular biomarkers identification and application in CHO processing. Journal of Biotechnology. 2024;**392**:11-24. DOI: 10.1016/j. jbiotec.2024

[3] Polissidis A, Lilian-Petropolou-Vathi MN-B, Rideout HJ. The future of targeted gene-based treatment strategies and biomarkers in Parkinson's disease. Biomolecules. 2020;**10**(6):912

[4] Grubb A, Löfberg H. Human gamma-trace, a basic microprotein; amino acid sequence and presence in the adenohypophysis. Proceedings of the National Academy of Sciences of the United States of America. 1982;**79**(9):3024-3027. Bibcode:1982PNAS. DOI: 10.1073/ pnas.70.9.3024

[5] Löfberg H, Grubb AO. Quantitation of gamma-trace in human biological fluids: Indications for production in the central nervous system. Scandinavian Journal of Clinical and Laboratory Investigation. 1979;**39**(7):619-626. DOI: 10.3109/00365517909108866

[6] Grubb A, Simonsen O, Sturfelt G, Truedsson L, Thysell H. Serum concentration of cystatin C, factor D and beta 2-microglobulin as a measure of glomerular filtration rate. Acta Medica Scandinavica. 1985;**218**(5):499-503. DOI: 10.1111/j.0954-6820.1985.tb08880.x

[7] Qiu X, Liu C, Ye Y, Li H, Chen Y, Fu Y, et al. The diagnostic value of serum creatinine and cystatin c in evaluating glomerular filtration rate in patients with chronic kidney disease: A systematic literature review and meta-analysis. Oncotarget. 2017;**8**(42):72985-72999. DOI: 10.18632/oncotarget.20271

[8] Masson I, Maillard N, Tack I, Thibaudin L, Dubourg L, Delanaye P, et al. GFR estimation using standardized cystatin C in kidney transplant recipients. American Journal of Kidney Diseases. 2013;**61**(2):279-284. DOI: 10.1053/j.ajkd.2012.09.010. Epub 2012 Nov 8. Erratum in: Am J Kidney Dis. Aug 2013;62(2):401

[9] Nakhjavan-Shahraki B, Yousefifard M, Ataei N, Baikpour M, Ataei F, Bazargani B, et al. Accuracy of cystatin C in prediction of acute kidney injury in children; serum or urine levels: Which one works better ? A systematic review and meta analysis. BMC Nephrology. 2017;**18**:1-20. DOI: 10.1186/ s12882-017-0539-0

[10] Benoit S, Ciccia EA, Devarajan P. Cystatin C as a biomarker of chronic kidney disease: Latest developments. Expert Review of Medicine Molecular Diagnostics. 2020;**20**(10):1019-1026. DOI: 10.1080/14737159.2020.1768849

[11] Jung E, Ro YS, Ryu HH, Kong SY, Do Shin S, Hwang SO. Cystatin C and mortality risk in the general population: Systematic review and dose response meta-analysis. Biomarkers. 2022;**27**(3):222-229. DOI: 10.1080/1354750X.2021.1989489

[12] Chen J, Yang Y, Dai C, Wang Y, Zeng R, Liu Q. Serum cystatin C is associated with the prognosis in acute myocardial infarction patients after coronary revascularization: A systematic review and meta-analysis.

BMC Cardiovascular Disorders. 2022;**22**:156. DOI: Doi.org/10.1186/s12872-022-02599-5

[13] Wang Y, Li W, Yang J, Zhang M, Tian C, Ma M, Zhang Q. Association Between Cystatin C and the Risk of Ischemic Stroke: A Systematic Review and Meta-analysis. Journal of Molecular Neuroscience. Nov 2019;**69**(3):444-449. DOI: 10.1007/s12031-019-01373-1. Epub 2019 Jul 17. PMID: 31313057

[14] Lafarge J-C, Naour N, Clement K, Guerre-Milo M. Cathepsins and cystatin C in atherosclerosis and obesity. Biochimie. 2010;**92**(11):1580-1586. DOI: 10.1016/j.biochi.2010.04.011

[15] Ma C-C, Duan C-C, Huang R-C, Tang H-Q. Association of circulating C levels with type 2 diabetes mellitus: A systematic review and meta-analysis. Archives of Medical Science. 2019;**16**(3):648-656. DOI: 10.5114/aoms.2019.83511

[16] Xin C, Xie J, Fan H, Sun X, Shi B. Association Between Serum Cystatin C and Thyroid Diseases: A Systematic Review and Meta-Analysis. Front Endocrinol (Lausanne). 19 Nov 2021;**12**:766516. DOI: 10.3389/fendo.2021.766516. PMID: 34867811; PMCID: PMC8639734

[17] Chai L, Feng W, Zhai C, Shi W, Wang J, Yan X, et al. The association between cystatinC and COPD: A meta-analysis and systematic review. BMC Pulmonary Medicine. 2020;**20**:182. DOI: doi.org/10.1186/s12890-020-01208-S

[18] Mathews PM, Levy E. Cystatin C in aging and in Alzheimer's disease. Ageing Research Reviews. 2016;**32**:38-50. DOI: 10.1016/j.arr.2016.06.003

[19] Ashrafian H, Zadeh EH, Khan RH. Review on Alzheimer's disease: Inhibition of amyloid beta and tau tangle formation. International Journal of Biological Macromolecules. 2021;**167**:382-394. DOI: 10.1016/j.ijbiomac.2020.11.192

[20] Nair P, Misra S, Nath M, Vibha D, Srivastava AK, Prasad K, et al. Cystatin C and risk of mild cognitive impairment: A systematic review and meta – Analysis. Dementia and Geriatric Cognitive Disorders. 2021;**49**(5):471-482. DOI: 10.1159/000510219

[21] Zinellu A, Mangoni AA. Cystatin C, COVID-19 severity and mortality: Asystematic review and meta-analysis. Journal of Nephrology. 2022;**35**:59-68. DOI: doi.org/10.1007/s40620-021-01139-2

[22] Leto G, Crescimanno M, Flandina C. On the role of cystatin C in cancer progression. Life Sciences. 2018;**202**:152-160. DOI: 10.1016/j.Ifs.2018.04.013

[23] Jiang Y, Zhang J, Zhang C, Hong L, Jiang Y, Ling L, et al. The role of cystatin C as a protcasomc inhibitor in multiple myeloma. Hematology. 2020;**5525**(1):457-463. DOI: 10.1080/16078454.2020.1850973

[24] Ding L, Liu Z, Wang J. Role of cystatin C in urogenital malignancy. Front Endocrinol (Lausanne). 14 Dec 2022;**13**:1082871. DOI: 10.3389/fendo.2022.1082871. PMID: 36589819; PMCID: PMC9794607

Chapter 2

# The Use of Cystatin C as a Marker of Glomerular Filtration Rate in Clinical Practice

*Flávia S. Reis and Elias David-Neto*

## Abstract

In the assessment of kidney function, it is widely acknowledged that the glomerular filtration rate (GFR) represents the most reliable indicator of kidney function. Ensuring precision and accuracy in the measurement (mGFR) or estimation of this GFR (eGFR) is of paramount importance. Cystatin C has emerged as a GFR marker, supported by scientific evidence. In addition to glomerular filtration, other variables or circumstances can influence the serum level of cystatin C, which is known as a non-GFR determinants. There has been discussion about the incorporation of race or genetic ancestry into eGFR. It is important to establish the role of cystatin C in this context, as well as in others involving the decision to use nonindexed eGFR, as well as the choice of the best tool for adjusting drug doses. Equations have been developed to estimate GFR using cystatin C, and the limitations and accuracy of these equations are presented here.

**Keywords:** cystatin C, estimated glomerular filtration rate, kidney function, creatinine, measured GFR

## 1. Introduction

The kidneys are responsible for maintaining the body's homeostasis by performing several functions, including the ability to filter the blood in a complex and highly selective process. The human kidney is comprised of approximately one million nephrons, which individually performs the filtration rate per nephron, defined as the volume of fluid filtered by a single nephron in a given time. This physiological process takes place in a network of capillaries, a structure known as the glomerulus or Malpighian corpuscles, first described by the Italian physician Marcelo Malpighi in 1662. It is generally accepted that the glomerular filtration rate (GFR) is the best index of kidney function that can be used in clinical practice. This is based on the premise that glomerular filtration is a primary and essential step for the kidneys to perform many regulatory functions. It is also accepted that with the loss of the ability to ultrafiltrate the blood, the other functions are also impaired. The average GFR in healthy young adults is around 120 mL/min/1.73m$^2$. This means that the 2 million nephrons together filter 172 liters of blood in a day or that the total plasma volume of an adult is filtered more than 50 times a day. It is not possible to measure the true glomerular filtration rate (tGFR) directly in humans, but it is possible to determine the clearance of certain molecules from the blood, known as measured GFR or mGFR method. There is a consensus that mGFR is the index that most closely approximates tGFR and is presented as the same measurement, although it is recognized that mGFR may not exactly match tGFR due to inherent variability in the kinetics of the exogenous marker used, the clearance method—whether renal or plasmatic—the mathematical model of plasma decay curves, and the laboratory tests used to quantify the exogenous marker. The renal inulin clearance method, originally described in 1935 by Homer W. Smith and James A. Shannon [1], remains the gold standard for measuring mGFR. With the development of simplified methods that show a high correlation with mGR by inulin, other exogenous markers have been used, including the radioisotopes $^{51}$Cr-EDTA, $^{99m}$Tc-DTPA, and $^{125}$I-iothalamate, as well as the contrast agents iohexol and iothalamate. Nevertheless, measuring GFR in a clinical context remains an impractical approach for sequential assessments and is still an expensive and inaccessible procedure limited to a few medical centers around the world. From an alternative and pragmatic perspective, GFR can be estimated (eGFR) by applying mathematical equations derived from the serum concentration of an endogenous marker such as cystatin C and creatinine. For almost a century [2], serum creatinine has been the primary marker of glomerular filtration, although it has its limitations in detecting early reductions in GFR. This is because creatinine levels do not rise until function has significantly deteriorated, that is, by about 50% [3]. These limitations are related to the variables that influence serum levels in addition to glomerular filtration and are referred to as non-GFR determinants. Cystatin C, a low-molecular-weight protein, has fewer non-GFR determinants than creatinine, and the performance of equations based on its serum concentration shows high accuracy compared to the reference mGFR used. Estimated GFR is critical in clinical practice for screening, staging and determining the prognosis of chronic kidney disease (CKD), assessing response to prescribed therapy, adjusting drug dosing, decision making for contrast testing, indication for dialysis therapy, or inclusion on the kidney transplant waiting list. This has prompted nephrologists and researchers to find an endogenous marker that enables an accurate estimation of GFR.

## 2. Cystatin C as an endogenous marker of GFR

The relationship between cystatin C and the glomerular filtration rate was first described in 1985 by Simonsen et al. [4]. In their study, which involved 106 patients, the inverse of the serum concentrations of cystatin C (ScysC) (r = 0.75), creatinine (Scr) (0.73), and β2-microglobulin (0.70) was closely correlated with the $^{51}$Cr-EDTA (mGFR), in contrast to the value for retinol-binding protein (r = 0.39). In the same year, Grubb et al. [5] conducted a similar study in 135 patients undergoing $^{51}$Cr-EDTA and found a correlation of 0.77, 0.75, 0.59, and 0.69 with cystatin C, creatinine, β2-microglobulin, and complement factor D, respectively. In their meta-analysis, Dharnidharka et al. [6] analyzed data from 54 studies with 4,492 participants and showed that ScysC is a more reliable indicator of glomerular filtration rate (GFR) than Scr. It is important to note that the studies at that time used the correlation coefficient or AUC analysis of the receiver operating characteristic curve (ROC) plot as a measure of the accuracy of the serum level of the marker. It was not until after the 2000s that a growing number of research studies were conducted to develop and evaluate the accuracy of cystatin C-based equations (eGFR-cysC) for estimating glomerular filtration rate. In addition, the analysis of isolated serum concentration is no longer the main focus. In 2002, the K/DOQI Clinical Practice Guidelines for Chronic Kidney Disease: Assessment, Classification, and Stratification [7] defined a metric standard based on the measurement bias as the median of the difference between the measured GFR (mGFR) and the estimated GFR (eGFR) and on the accuracy at P30 (>90%) and at P10, that is, the percentage of eGFR estimates that fall within the interval mGFR±30% and the interval mGFR±10%, respectively. This approach was then used by most subsequent studies and standardization of metrics was a crucial aspect to facilitate comparisons between studies. Moreover, the introduction of international certification for cystatin C assays in 2010 by the Working Group for the Manufacture of an International Cystatin C Calibrator (WG-SCC) enabled various diagnostic companies to produce cystatin C assays with less inter-assay variability and supported the standardization of the measurement of ScysC and the comparability of results between studies [8]. The first recommendation for the use of cystatin C in a medical guideline was in the KDIGO 2012 Clinical Practice Guidelines for the Assessment and Treatment of Chronic Kidney Disease [9], which included the recommendation to measure cystatin C as a confirmatory test with an eGFRcr of 45-59 mL/min/1.73 m$^2$ without markers of kidney impairment such as albuminuria when confirmation of CKD is required. In 2024, an update to this guideline [10] reaffirms the use of cystatin C in the diagnostic assessment of CKD, which includes an eGFR with both markers, cystatin C, and creatinine (eGFRcysC-cr), which has significant prognostic implications when cystatin C is added to the initial assessment of these patients. One of the biggest barriers to greater accessibility and widespread use of cystatin C is the cost of the reagents, which is about $5 per test, compared to about $0.50 per test for sCr in the US, although the laboratory's operating costs are similar to those for creatinine; another barrier is the difficulty in obtaining reimbursement given the conditions imposed by health insurance companies. In 2020, Medicare reimbursement was $5.12 and $18.52 for creatinine and cystatin C, respectively [11]. It is reasonable to predict that the cost of the reagents will tend to decrease as knowledge of cystatin C spreads in the medical community and the number of medical requests for the test increases.

The following sessions provide an in-depth account of the knowledge accrued over the past years that has led to the establishment of cystatin C as an accurate marker of glomerular filtration rate. A bibliographic search was carried out in the PubMed database using the main terms cystatin C and glomerular filtration rate.

## 3. The molecular properties of cystatin C make it an effective GFR marker

Cystatin C is a non-glycosylated protein with a molecular weight of 13.35 kDa and an isoelectric point of 9.3. The cystatin C gene is expressed in all nucleated cells that exhibit stable cystatin C production, resulting in a constant steady-state serum level. The protein is secreted into extracellular fluids [12]. It was originally identified by Jorgen Clausen as a gamma globulin in cerebrospinal fluid [13] and by Butler and Flynn as a protein with a post-gamma electrophoretic profile found in urine samples from 46 patients with kidney disease, including eight patients with Fanconi syndrome [14]. The low weight and positive charge of cystatin C allows its passage through the glomerular filtration membrane, a structure composed of three main components, the endothelial cell, the basement membrane, and the podocyte with its "slit membranes," which has a size selectivity for molecules and contains proteoglycans, glycosaminoglycans, and collagens which confer an electrostatic barrier property that repels negatively charged proteins. Molecules close to the size of inulin (molecular weight 5.2 kDa) are filtered freely, while others, such as myoglobin (molecular weight 17 kDa), are filtered to a lesser extent than inulin and albumin (molecular weight 69 kDa), which is practically not filtered. After ultrafiltration, cystatin C is reabsorbed by the proximal tubule cell through its direct binding to megalin, an endocytic receptor in the apical membrane, and is subsequently completely degraded in the lysozomes, so does not return to the circulation in its native form [15, 16]. Significant amounts of cystatin C are not expected to be present in the urine under physiological conditions. Therefore, it is not possible to evaluate the renal clearance of cystatin C in the same way as the renal clearance of creatinine. The above description fulfills many of the criteria for an ideal filtration marker, which to date has been attributed to inulin, a fructose polymer with a molecular weight of 5.2 kDa that does not bind to plasma proteins, is distributed in the extracellular fluid, is freely filtered by the glomeruli, and is neither reabsorbed nor secreted by the renal tubule cell. Furthermore, an ideal marker is defined by the fact that it appears in the plasma at a constant rate from an endogenous source. This is a property that inulin as an exogenous molecule does not possess, but cystatin C does. The question is whether the concentration of cystatin C in the blood is always constant or whether certain clinical conditions can disrupt its production rate, which will be presented in the next session.

## 4. Non-GFR determinants that may influence the serum level of cystatin C

It is therefore essential that clinicians are aware of the variable non-glomerular filtration rate (non-GFR) in order to correctly interpret serum values and GFR estimates from endogenous markers. Cystatin C production appears to be more uniform in different populations than creatinine production, which has been shown to exhibit considerable heterogeneity due to variables unrelated to glomerular filtration [17]. After adjusting for mGFR, cystatin C is less influenced by age, gender, ethnicity, muscle mass, protein intake, renal tubule management, and extrarenal elimination compared to creatinine. However, cystatin C has other factors that are not related to GFR. This section provides an overview of the key issues and questions that have been explored in the current literature, summarized in **Figure 1**.

Serum creatinine levels increase in proportion to muscle mass, which is influenced by various factors such as gender, ethnicity, age, general health status, and dietary protein intake. In addition to the factors related to the generation of creatinine, there are also physiological processes related to the excretion of creatinine by tubular and extra-renal secretion through the gastrointestinal tract. In one of the first studies to examine these non-GFR variables, Knight et al. [18] found in a cross-sectional analysis of the Prevention of Renal and Vascular End-Stage Disease (PREVEND) cohort (n = 8,058 patients) that older age, male sex, higher weight, taller height, current cigarette smoking, and higher serum C-reactive protein (CRP) levels were independently associated with higher serum cystatin C levels; however, the fact that these variables were adjusted for creatinine clearance and not a mGFR limited the interpretation of these results. Using a pooled dataset of four studies (n = 3,418 patients) and GFR measured by [125]I-iothalamate or [51]Cr-EDTA, Stevens et al. [19] showed a stronger association of serum creatinine than cystatin C with surrogates of

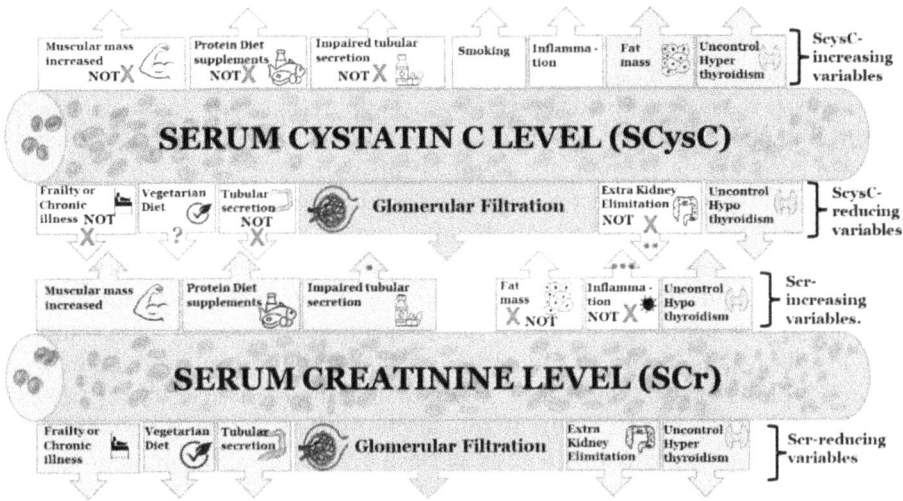

**Figure 1.**
*Non-GFR determinants for cystatin C and creatinine. ? Not known. NOT ✕: variable that does not affect the serum level of the marker. * Impairment of tubular secretion by drugs such as cimetidine, trimethoprim, fenofibrate, dolutegravir. ** It appears that extrarenal elimination is negligible in rats with intact kidneys when considering the renal plasma clearance of $^{125}I$-cystatin C compared to the clearance of $^{51}Cr$-EDTA. *** If inflammation is a causal factor in chronic illness, it can lead to a reduction in serum creatinine level.*

muscle mass, including age, sex, ethnicity, and urine creatinine. Subsequently, Liu et al. [20] in a pooled cross-sectional analysis of three studies involving 3,156 individuals with chronic kidney disease in which GFR was measured found that creatinine was more strongly associated with male sex, Black ethnicity, larger body surface area, taller height, and higher urine creatinine than cystatin C and β2 microglobulin (β2m); and that cystatin C and creatinine had no strong associations in common; however, both β2m and cystatin C, but not creatinine, had an intermediate association with smoking. One year later, Foster et al. [21] in a cross-sectional analysis from the Age, Gene/Environment Susceptibility Kidney Study (AGES-Kidney; n = 683 patients) and from the Multi-Ethnic Study of Atherosclerosis Kidney Study (MESA-Kidney; n = 275) found that estimated GFR by cystatin C, β2m, and beta trace protein (BTP) had significantly less strong residual associations with age and gender than eGFR by creatinine and was not associated with ethnicity (Black vs. White) in MESA-Kidney; eGFRcys and eGFRβ2m, but not eGFR-BTP, showed significant residual associations with C-reactive protein levels in both studies. In a cross-sectional analysis from the Renal Iohexol Clearance Survey Study, Schei et al. [22] examined 1,627 patients without kidney disease, diabetes, or cardiovascular disease. They found that both eGFRcr and eGFRcysC were associated with inflammatory markers after adjustment of mGFR by iohexol, but in opposite directions. While the aforementioned cohort studies found an association between serum levels of cystatin C and C-reactive protein, this association was not confirmed by other study designs [23, 24]. Grubb et al. [25] conducted individual studies on patients undergoing elective surgery. They observed a significant increase in the initial inflammatory marker, which reached maximum levels on the second postoperative day, and found no correlation with ScysC levels. A significant correlation between the ScysC level and body mass index (BMI) has been documented [18, 26]. Chew-Harris et al. [27] found that body composition, particularly body fat as determined by bioelectrical impedance (BIA) and dual-energy X-ray absorptiometry (DEXA), correlated significantly with ScysC level. In the multiple regression analysis, only fat mass and mGFR using $^{99m}$Tc-DTPA were identified as independent factors influencing cystatin C. On the other hand, age and skeletal muscle mass were identified as the most important determinants of creatinine in this model. A comparable correlation was found by Naour et al. [28] in their analysis of cystatin C in 237 non-obese and 248 obese participants and in a special subgroup of patients from a gastrosurgery program. Subcutaneous and visceral tissue biopsies from obese subjects showed a threefold increase in mRNA expression of cystatin C, with comparable levels observed in omental and subcutaneous adipose tissue from the same individual. From these studies, it can be deduced that adipose tissue plays at least some part in the increase in serum concentrations of cystatin C (ScysC) in obese individuals. One hypothesis is that this increased production of cystatin C represents a protective mechanism that regulates the activity of cathepsins associated with atherosclerosis and inflammation. Administration of high doses of steroids was also associated with an increase in cystatin C, a phenomenon that appears to be dose-dependent [29]. This effect has been specifically associated with methylprednisolone pulses [30] and is not reproducible with the standard doses of steroids commonly used [31]. In HeLa cell cultures, Bjarnadottir et al. [32] observed a stronger secretion of cystatin C after dexamethasone, a dose-dependent effect. This suggests that the increase in production is due to the increased expression of the cystatin C gene. Thyroid dysfunction has been identified as a transient modifier of cystatin C production, with a significant increase or decrease in serum levels observed in uncontrol hyperthyroidism and hypothyroidism, respectively. It is reasonable to assume that this finding can be attributed to changes in cell turnover and metabolism. Once normal hormone levels are restored (euthyroid state), the serum cystatin C level returns to its baseline value. Serum creatinine levels show the opposite effect, falling or rising in uncontrol hyperthyroidism and hypothyroidism, respectively. This is attributed to the known influence of thyroid hormones on renal hemodynamics and tubular transport [33, 34].

## 5. Performance of equations to estimate GFR from serum cystatin C

As mentioned above, the serum concentration of an endogenous marker of renal function is primarily determined by glomerular filtration, and the two are inversely related. It should be noted that other processes can also influence the formation or clearance of the molecule, both renal and extra-renal, which are referred to as factors unrelated to glomerular filtration or non-GFR determinants. These factors lead to a reduction in the accuracy of the serum concentration of the endogenous marker when used as an index of renal function. The inclusion of demographic and clinical variables as surrogates for non-GFR determinants, such as gender, age, and ethnicity, serves to mitigate the effects of these factors according to their relationship to each other, thus improving accuracy compared to the serum marker value alone. There are additional sources of error in the estimation of GFR, including systematic differences between the populations in which the equation was developed, the population in which it was validated, and the population in which it is applied in clinical practice, as these factors of non-GFR vary across populations, and furthermore, there are differences in the methods used to assess mGFR and in laboratory testing of endogenous markers, which are employed in the models used to develop the equation. It is important to be aware of these aspects in order to correctly interpret the GFR estimates derived from the equations and to select the most appropriate equation for clinical practice.

## 5.1 Cystatin C equations

Over the last two decades, various equations have been developed to estimate GFR based on ScysC and demographic variables. These equations are listed in **Tables 1-3**. For adults, one of the first formulas was proposed by Hoek et al. [39] based on a sample of 93 patients undergoing urinary clearance of $^{125}$I-iothalamate and $^{131}$I-hippuran and a 2-year longitudinal analysis of 30 diabetic patients. Cystatin C results began to become abnormal near the mGFR cut-off level of 90 mL/min/1.73m², while creatinine levels were still within the normal reference range and maintained significant differences between the two markers until the mGFR cut-off level of 60 mL/min/1.73m² was reached. The first equation to use the standardized cystatin C value was the Chronic Kidney Disease Epidemiology Collaboration (CKDEPI-2012), which used the variables such as gender and age without taking ethnicity into account. Additionally, in the same study, the combined equation with the creatinine and cystatin C markers was also expressed, called the CKDEPI 2012 creatinine-cystatin C equation (CKDEPIcr-cysC), with the variables such as sex, age, and race, but with a lower race correction factor than that previously proposed in the CKDEPI 2009 if Black race was self-reported, the correction factor was 1.08 and 1.159, respectively [36, 53]. The combined equation has performed better in many studies, as shown in **Table 2**. The CAPA equation was developed by Grubb et al. [42] in 2014 from a sample of 4,960 participants from comprising Caucasian, Asian, Pediatric, and Adult participants (CAPA) cohort to evaluate the concordance in the estimation of eGFR-cysC after efforts to optimize and certify six commercially available cystatin C assays. The CAPA equation does not include coefficients for ethnicity or sex and is therefore virtually assay independent.

In 2021, the CKDEPI equations were reissued without the ethnicity variable [45], as described in Section 5.4 below. In brief, the CKDEPIcr 2021 update excludes the ethnicity variable but still requires the gender variable to account for discrepancies between male and female populations, and had lower performance compared to the CKDEPIcreat2009 equation in White European populations, and only partial performance improvements were observed in Black Europeans and Black Africans. The CKDEPIcr and CKDEPIcr-cysC 2021 equations were immediately endorsed by the American Society of Nephrology and the National Kidney Foundation in the USA, while the European Federation of Clinical Chemistry and Laboratory Medicine (EFLM) did not recommend it and instead suggested the newer equation developed by the European Kidney Function Consortium (EKFC). The EKFCcysC [40] equation is based on cystatin C and has the same mathematical equation as the EKFC equation based on creatinine [54]. It simply replaces the scaled creatinine with the scaled cystatin C and determines the "Q-value" factor based on the median SCysC level in a healthy population across the age spectrum (transition from children to adults and from adults to the elderly). The eGFR-EKFCcr divides the serum creatinine level by the median serum creatinine level of healthy participants, controlling for the non-GFR determinants of age, gender, and ethnicity. The value of the scaling Q-factor for cystatin C was set at 0.83 for men and women under 50 years of age and 0.83 + 0.005 x (age − 50) for those over 50 years of age. This is based on data from 227,643 White patients in Sweden. This Q value for cystatin C does not vary by gender or ethnicity. Then, the EKFC$_{CysC}$ can be used independently of gender and race.

| Equation Y/ authors | Stand. assay / continent | CysC equation | mGFR | Sample size/population | Comments/main results |
|---|---|---|---|---|---|
| **Adults** | | | | | |
| Japanese 2013; Horio et al. [35] | Yes/ Asian | eGFR (mL/min/1.73 m²) = 96 x SCysC$^{-1.324}$ x 0.996$^{Age}$ x 0.894 (if female) | Inulin (ur) | n = 413 and N = 350 in the development and validation datasets | Favorable for CKDEPI$_{CysC2012}$ |
| CKD-EPI$_{2012}$ 2012 Inker et al. [36] | Yes/ North American (USA) | Female or male; SCysC ≤ 0.80: $133 \times (SCysC/0.80)^{-0.499} \times 0.9962^{age}$ [x 0.932 if female]; SCysC > 0.80: $133 \times (SCysC/0.80)^{-1.328} \times 0.9962^{age}$ [x 0.932 if female] | Iothal. (ur) | n = 5352 from 13 studies (development and internal)—33% Black; n = 1119 (the external validation) | eGFRcr and eGFR cysC have similar accuracy. Favorable $_{eGFRcr\_CysC\,2012}$ |
| Stevens et al. 2008 [37] | No/ USA and European | eGFR1 = 76.7 x cystatin C (mg/L)$^{-1.19}$; eGFR2 = 127.7 x cystatin C (mg/L)$^{-1.17}$ x age$^{-0.13}$ x (0.91 if female) x (1.06 if Black) | $^{51}$CrEDTA (ur) or Iothl. (ur) | n = 2980 three CKD studies in the US (MDRD, ASK, and CSG) n = 438, from Paris | Compared with MDRD; favorable for eGFRcr-cysC |
| RULE et al. [38] 2006 | No/ European, Sweden | eGFR = 66.8 x cystatin C (mg/L)$^{-1.30}$ | Iothal. (ur) | n = 460 (42% female; 97% Caucasian; mean age of 51 ± 15 y) | eGFRcysC $r^2 = 0.853$ eGFRcr $r^2 = 0.827$ |
| HOEK et al. [39] 2003 | No/ European, Amsterdam | eGFR = 80.35/cystatin C (mg/L)—4.32 | $^{125}$I-Iothal. 131 I-Hippu | n = 93 several diseases n = 30 with diabetes age 50 years (11–77) | eGFRcysC bias: −2.4 ± 12.09 vs. +15.9 ± 15.41 C&G |
| **Adults and children** | | | | | |
| EKFC 2023 Pottel et al. [40] | Yes/North European (only White European in the development dataset) | The general form of the EKFC eGFR equation is: eGFR-EKFC = 107.3/[Biomarker/Q]$^{\alpha}$ x [0.990$^{(Age-40)}$ if age > 40 years], with α = 0.322 when biomarker/Q is less than 1 and α = 1.132 when biomarker/Q is 1 or more. | $^{51}$Cr-EDTA or$^{99}$Tc-DTPA or inulin/ Ioh. or Iothal. | n = 7727 White EKFC Coh./ n = 2646 White n = 858 Black from Paris coh/ n = 1093 White US coh./n = 508 Black/ African | EFKCcysC not better EFKCcr, but better than CKDEPI2021 Favorable for EFKC$_{cr-cysC}$ |
| FAS$_{cysC}$ Pottel et al. 2017 [41] | Yes/ European | FAScysC = 107.3 / (ScysC/QcysC) X [0.988 $^{(Age-40)}$ when age > 40 years | $^{51}$CrEDTA or Inulin or Ioh. or Iothal. | n = 6132 (368 children; 4295 adult and 1469 older adult ≥70 years); only White | Favorable for FAS $_{Cr\_CysC}$ and CKDEPI$_{cr\_CysC}$ and BIS2 (cr-cysC) |

| Equation Y/ authors | Stand. assay / continent | CysC equation | mGFR | Sample size/population | Comments/main results |
|---|---|---|---|---|---|
| CAPA 2014 Grubb et al. [42] | Yes / European/ Asian | $eGFR = 130 \times cysC^{-1.069} \times age^{-0.117} - 7$ | Inulin (pl or ur) Iohe. (pl) | n = 3495 Swedish (Lund CysC stand. Cohort – LCS) n = 763 Japanese adults/ n = 702 childr. | CAPA does not require a sex or race factor; interassay CV was 2,8% |
| GRUBB et al. [43] 2005 | No/ European, Sweden | $eGFR = 84.69c$ cystatin C $(mg/L)^{-1.680}$ (x1.384 if child <14 years) | Iohe. (pl) | n = 536 (451 adults/32 children 14–17 years and 53 was 0.3–13 y) | eGFRcys $r^2 = 0.805$ eGFR Schwartz $r^2 = 0.761$ |
| LARSSON et al. [44] 2004 | No/ Sweden European | $eGFR = 77.239 \times$ cystatin C $(mg/L)^{-21.2623}$ | Iohe. (pl) | n = 100 (40fem/60 mal.); age 4–92 y | eGFRcysCr$^2 = 0.910$ eGFRcr $r^2 = 0.840$ |

Y: year. Stand: Standardization assay. EKFC: European Kidney Function Consortium; FAS: full age spectrum; CKD-EPI: chronic kidney disease epidemiology collaboration; MDRD: modification of diet in renal disease equation created in 1999 for estimated GFR. AASK: African American Study of Kidney Disease; CSG: Collaborative Study Group. C&G—Cockcroft &Gault equation (The formula was created in 1976 and is based on creatinine for the estimation of creatinine clearance; however, it does not estimate GFR). Iohe: Iohexol; pl.: plasmatic clearance; Iothal: Iothalamate; ur: urinary clearance; bias (mL/min/1.73m²): the median of the difference between measured GFR and estimated GFR.

**Table 1.**
eGFR based on cystatin C levels in adults and children.

| Equation/ authors/ year | Stand. assay | CysC equation | mGFR | Sample size/population |
|---|---|---|---|---|
| **Adult** | | | | |
| CKD-EPI$_{cys C, cr}$ Inker et al. [45] 2021 | Yes/ | eGFR = 135 X min(Scr/κ,1)$^\alpha$ X max(Scr/κ,1) $^{-0.544}$ X min(Scys/0.8,1) $^{-0.323}$ X max(Scys/0.8,1) $^{-0.778}$ X 0.9961$^{Age}$ X 0.963 [if female] κ = 0.7 (females) or 0.9 (males) α = −0.219 (females) or − 0.144 (males) min = indicates the minimum of SCr/κ or 1 max = indicates the maximum of SCr/κ or 1. * Scr mg/dL. ScysC mg/L | Iothal. (ur)/ $^{51}$CrEDTA and Iohe. | n = 8254 (from CKDEPI2009) n = 5352 (from CKDEPI2012) n = 4050 for validation |
| Japanese 2013 Horio et al. [35] | Yes | eGFR = 92 × Cystatin C$^{-0.575}$ × Creatinine $^{-0.670}$ × 0.995$^{Age}$ × 0.784 [if female] | Inulin (ur) | n = 413 and n = 350 in the development and validation |
| CKD-EPI$_{cys C, cr}$ Inker et al. [36] 2012 | Yes | eGFR = 135 × min(Scr/κ, 1)$^\alpha$ × max(Scr/κ, 1) $^{-0.601}$ × min(Scys/0.8, 1) $^{-0.375}$ × max(Scys/0.8, 1) $^{-0.711}$ × 0.995$^{Age}$ [× 0.969 if female] [× 1.08 if Black] where Scr is serum creatinine, Scys is serum cystatin C, κ is 0.7 for females and 0.9 for males, α is −0.248 for females and − 0.207 for males, min indicates the minimum of Scr/κ or 1, and max indicates the maximum of Scr/κ or 1. | $^{125}$I-Iothal. (ur) | n = 5352 from 13 studies (development and internal validation; 33% Black) n = 1119 (the external validation) |
| Stevens [37] eGFR$_{cr, cysC}$ 2008 | No | eGFR3 = 177.6 x plasma creatinine/88.4 (mmol/L) $^{-0.65}$ x cystatin C (mg/L) $^{-0.57}$ x age $^{-0.20}$ x (0.82 if female) x (1.11 if Black) | $^{51}$CrEDTA (ur) or Iothl. (ur) | n = 2980 three CKD studies in the US (MDRD, ASK, and CSG) n = 438, from Paris (validation) |
| **Adult and children** | | | | |
| EKFC eGFR$_{cysC, cr}$ Pottel et al. [40] 2023 | Yes | The general form of the EKFC eGFR equation is: eGFR-EKFC = 107.3/[Biomarker/Q]$^\alpha$ × [0.990$^{(Age−40)}$ if age > 40 years], with α = 0.322 when biomarker/Q is less than 1 and α = 1.132 when biomarker/Q is 1 or more. | $^{51}$CrEDTA or Iohe. or $^{99}$Tc-DTPA or Inulin or Iothal | n = 7727 White/ EKFC Coh. n = 2646 (White = 858 Black from Paris cohort / n = 1093 White/US coh. n = 508 Black/ African coh) |
| FAS$_{comb(cys C, cr)}$ Pottel et al. [41] 2017 | Yes | $$FAScysC = \frac{107.3}{\alpha \times (Scr/Qcr) + (1-\alpha) \times (ScysC/QcysC)}$$ X [0.988 $^{(Age−40)}$ when age > 40 years] | $^{51}$CrEDTA or Inulin or Iohe. or Iothal. | n = 6132 (368 children; 4295 adult and 1469 older adult ≥70 y only White participants from 11 cohorts) |

| Equation/ authors/ year | Stand. assay | CysC equation | | mGFR | Sample size/population |
|---|---|---|---|---|---|
| | | Males | Females | | |
| **Children** | | | | | |
| Quadratic formula Crea_CysC Chehade et al. [46] 2014 | Yes | $0.42 \times (Ht = SCrea) - 0.04 \times (ht/SCrea)^2 - 14.5 \times ScysC + 0.69 \times age + 21.88$ | $0.42 \times (Ht = SCrea) - 0.04 \times (ht/SCrea)^2 - 14.5 \times ScysC + 0.69 \times age + 18.25$ | Inulin (ur) | n = 238 mean age: 12 ± 4.1 years P30: 97% |
| | | Ht is in cm, Screa in mg/dL, ScysC ir: mg/L and age in years | | | |
| Schwartz CKiD Cr_cysC updating 2012 [47] | No | $eGFR = 39.8 \times [height/SCr(mg/dL)]^{0.456} \times [1.8/ScysC(mg/L)]^{0.418} \times [30/BUN(mg/dL)]^{0.079} \times [1.076]^{gender} \times [height/1.4]^{0.179}$ | | Iohexol (pl) | n = 965 person-visits (1/3 as a validation dataset) |
| Schwartz CKiD Cr_cysC 2009 [48] | No | $eGFR = 39.1[height/Scr]^{0.516}[1.8/SCysC]^{0.294} \times [30/BUN]^{0.169}[1.099]^{male}[height/1.4]^{0.188}$ | | Iohexol (pl) | n = 349 children (61% female, 69% White, 15% Black) |
| Zappitelli 2006 Cyst_Crea eq Zappitelli et al. [49] | No | $GFR\ (mL/min/1.73\ m^2) = (43.82 \times e^{0.003 \times height}) / (SCysC^{0.635} \times SCr^{0.547}$ If renal transplant, $\times 1.165$ If spina bifida, $\times 1.57\ xSCr^{0.925}$ | | [125]I-Iothal (pl) | n = 103 children (60% male) mean age of 12.7 ± 4.7 years, North American, Canada |

*Stand: Standardization assay. EKFC: European Kidney Function Consortium. CKDEPI: Chronic Kidney Disease Epidemiology Collaboration equation. Iohe: Iohexol; pl.: plasmatic clearance; Iothal: Iothalamate; ur: urinary clearance; bias (mL/min/1.73m$^2$): the median of the difference between measured GFR and estimated GFR.*

**Table 2.**
*eGFR on the basis of cystatin C and creatinine combined equations.*

| Equation/ Authors/Year | Stand. Assay/C | CysC equation | mGFR | Sample size/ | Comments/ main results |
|---|---|---|---|---|---|
| CKiD eGFR CysC U25 2021 Pierce et al. [50] where 25 refers to age in years | Yes/ North American | $eGFR = K \times 1/ScysC$ (mg/L); K value, according to age and gender: <br><br> **Males**     **Females** <br> For 1 to <15   1 to <12 <br> $y = 87.2x1.011^{(age-15)}$   $y = 79.9x1.004^{(age-12)}$ <br> 15 to <18y = $872x0.960^{(age-15)}$   12 to <br> For 18 to 25 y = 77.1   $18y = 79.9x0.974^{(age-12)}$ <br> 18 to 25 y = 68.3 | Iohe. (pl) | n = 1093 person-visits from 387 males; n = 71 person-visits from 231 females 1/5 Black race | Improves performance vs. "bedside CysC" 2012 |
| Schwartz et al. CKiD CysC "bedside"cysC 2012 [47] | No/ North American | $eGFR = 70.69 \times [ScysC\ (mg/L)] - 0.931$ | Iohe. (pl) | n = 643 (254 girls; 389 boys)/ n = 322 (validation) | CKiD bias +0.3 mL P30:82.6% |
| Zappitelli CysC eq [49] 2006 | No/ North American (Canada) | $GFR\ (mL/min/1.73\ m^2) = 75.94/[ScysC^{1.17}]$ If renal transplant, x 1.2 <br> *ScysC in mg/L | $^{125}$I-Iothal. (pl) | n = 103 children (60% boys) mean age: 12.7 ± 4.7 y | Mean Bias eGFRCys: −1.2 (−4.4 – +2.3) Schwartz +6.9 (+2.3 – +11.6) |
| Filler & Lepage [51] 2003 | No/ North American (Canada) | $eGFR = 1.962 + [1.123x\log(1/ScysC)]$ | $^{99}$Tc-DTPA (pl) | n = 536/ 41% girls age: 1–18 y | Favorable to eGFRCys (Bias: +0.3%) vs. eGFR Schwartz (Bias: +10.8%) |
| Bokenkamp et al. [52] 1998 | No/ European Hannover | $eGFRCysC\ [mL/min/1.73\ m^2] = 162/ScysC[mg/L] - 30$ | Inulin (ur) | n = 87 girls 97 boys | eGFRcysC: bias: + 2.37 1/ScysC r = 0.88 |

Stand: Standardization assay; C: Continent; mGFR: measured GFR; CKiD: Chronic Kidney Disease in children prospective cohort study. Iohe: Iohexol; pl.: plasmatic clearance; Iothal: Iothalamate; ur: urinary clearance; bias (mL/min/1.73 m²): the median of the difference between measured GFR and estimated GFR; P30: as the proportion of patients with an estimated glomerular filtration rate (eGFR) that is within 30% of the measured GFR.

**Table 3.**
eGFR based on cystatin C levels in children and adolescents.

An important and vulnerable aspect of clinical practice is the identification of individuals with chronic kidney disease (CKD). A substantial body of evidence supports the accuracy of eGFRcysC in correctly classifying CKD stages and in risk stratification for adverse outcomes. In a meta-analysis of 90,750 participants from 11 studies in the general population and 2,960 participants with CKD from 5 studies, Shlipak et al. [55] documented a higher prevalence of CKD by eGFRcysC than by eGFRcr (13.7 vs. 9.7%) in the general population. The strongest association was observed between the risk of death from any cause and eGFRcysC, with a stronger correlation than with eGFRcr or eGFRcr-cysC. In addition, an important finding was the marked reverse J-shaped association observed with eGFRcr, which may be attributed to non-GFR determinants of creatinine known to be present in the chronically ill individuals, with an increased risk of death. Regarding cardiovascular mortality, the thresholds for a significant increase in risk were 69 mL/min/1.73m$^2$ for eGFRcr, 86 mL/min/1.73m$^2$ for eGFRcysC, and 83 mL/min/1.73m$^2$ for eGFRcysC-cr. In a prospective study with a follow-up of 4.6 years and 26,643 adult participants from the Reasons for Geographic and Racial Differences in Stroke (REGARDS) cohort study, Peralta et al. [56] investigated the effectiveness of a triple approach (eGFR-CKDEPIcr, eGFR-CKDEPIcysc, and urinary albumin-to-creatinine ratio [ACR]) in improving the detection of risks associated with CKD compared with creatinine alone. The inclusion of eGFR-CKDEPIcysC in the CKD detection model resulted in 5.2% of the cohort being reclassified to a higher risk group. This group had a threefold higher mortality rate (10% during follow-up) and a nearly fourfold higher risk of end-stage renal disease (0.62%) than those whose risk was reduced by the addition of eGFR-CKDEPIcysC (0.15%). In 2022, Chen et al. [57] conducted an analysis of 4,956 participants in the Chronic Renal Insufficiency Cohort (CRIC STUDY). The aim of the analysis was to assess the extent of discrepancies in the measurement of eGFRcr and eGFRcysC in relation to the risk of end-stage kidney disease (ESKD) and mortality in a population with chronic kidney disease (CKD). Compared to participants in whom eGFRcysC and eGFRcr were similar, those with eGFRcys lower than eGFRcr had a higher risk of ESKD and mortality. Conversely, those with eGFRcysC higher than eGFRcr had a lower risk of these outcomes. In longitudinal analyses, participants whose eGFRcysC decreased faster than eGFRcr had an 8.2-fold higher risk of death than participants in whom the difference between eGFRcr and eGFRcysC remained unchanged over time. In general, it can be inferred that a percentage of individuals at high risk of CKD are not identified as having CKD by eGFRcr alone. However, they are identified by eGFRcysC or even eGFRcysC-cr. These results also show the importance of monitoring cystatin C throughout patient follow-up.

## 5.2 Cystatin C and creatinine combined equations

Recent cohort studies on the development and validation of equations using creatinine and cystatin C simultaneously in populations with comorbidities show better performance than when using eGFRcr or eGFRcysC alone. This could be due to the fact that these markers do not have the same non-GFR determinants or are at least partially independent of each other, so simultaneous use reduces the errors associated with each marker individually. Adingwupu et al. [58] conducted a systematic review that included 26 studies published between 2011 and 2023. The studies assessed mGFR and used a standardized assay for laboratory cystatin C and creatinine measurement in clinical populations with cancer, HIV, cirrhosis and liver transplant, heart failure, neuromuscular disease, and obesity. The results showed a favorable outcome for the equations that employed the simultaneous use of both markers (eGFRcysC-cr) in populations with HIV, cancer, and obesity, supporting the use of combined equations in this clinical setting. **Table 2** illustrates the main equations applicable when creatinine and cystatin C markers are used simultaneously. Fu et al. [59] conducted a study to compare the CKDEPI and EKFC equations. The study included 6,174 participants from the Stockholm Creatinine Measurements (SCREAM) project. These participants had their mGFR determined by Iohexol plasma clearance between January 2011 and December 2021. This resulted in a total of 9,579 mGFR measurements. The study population had a high prevalence of comorbidities, including cardiovascular disease (30%), liver disease (28%), diabetes (26%), and cancer (26%). All eGFRcysC equations showed minimal bias: 0.8 for CKD-EPIcysC 2012, 2.5 for CKD-EPIcysC 2021, 1.0 for EKFCcysC, and − 1.5 mL/min/1.73m$^2$ for the mean of RLM/CAPA equation. However, after evaluating all metrics together, the combined equations eGFRcr-CysC showed the best performance with an accuracy of 88 to 91% (P30) and a bias of −1.5 to +2.5 mL/min/1.73m$^2$.

### 5.3 A single equation that can be applied to all age groups

In general, GFR estimation is calculated using a specific equation for children and adolescents, adults, and the elderly. In 2005, Grubb et al. [43] introduced the concept of a single equation for all age groups based on cystatin C, shown in **Table 1**. Pottel et al. [60] expanded this concept in 2016 with the introduction of the Full Age Spectrum (FAS) equation, which is based on three fundamental principles. (1) Population-normalized creatinine, referred to as Scr/Qcr; (2) GFR begins to decline around age 40; and (3) the average GFR for a healthy population 2 years of age and older is 107.3 mL/min/1.73m$^2$. The FAScr does not require adjustment for gender and age, in addition to proposing to resolve the discontinuity between the child/adolescent/adult and adult/elderly phases. Prior to 2016, the most commonly used equations in adults were the CKDEPI equations, while in children the Schwartz equation was the predominant choice and in older people the CKDEPI equations or Berlin Initiative Study (BIS) equations. The latter will be discussed in more detail in Section 7. In 2017, the FAScysC versions and FAScysC-cr were edited with both markers using data from the same population and following the same principles as the FAScr version and are presented in **Tables 1** and **2**. In pediatric populations, the combined FAS equation demonstrated a P30 of 92.1%, which surpassed the performance of eGFR-CAPA and eGFR-Schwarts-CysC in a validation study of 6,132 participants. In the elderly, the combined FAS equation showed comparable performance to the combined BIS (BIS2) equation and had higher accuracy compared to the CKDEPI-cysC and CKDEPI-cr-cysC-2012 equations. In adults, the performance of the FAS equations in both versions was comparable to that of the CKDEPI equations [41]. The EKFC equation, referenced in Section 5.1 above, represents an advancement of the Full Age Spectrum method and both provide an accurate estimate of GFR in pediatric, adult, and older populations and are a valuable and attractive approach, particularly in individual Caucasian descent.

### 5.4 Estimating GFR by cystatin C without race

Race is a variable that more strongly influences estimates of GFR from creatinine, possibly associated with non-GFR determinants of the creatinine, which may vary between ethnicities. When developing equations, a calibration factor is usually required to improve the accuracy of the estimate by creatinine (eGFRcr). In Asian populations, the use of equations based on creatinine also requires an adjustment coefficient, which is not required for equations based on ScysC level [35]. In general, equations based on ScysC level exhibit greater accuracy in Asian population [61]. It is known that serum creatinine (Scr) levels are higher in Black people compared to other ethnic groups within the same mGFR measurement range. This is the reason for including ethnicity in this GFR estimate; otherwise, mGFR would be underestimated in Black people. Consequently, the estimated GFR values are higher when Black ethnicity is reported in the electronic medical calculators accessible on applications and websites. In the 2009 CKDEPI equation, which included 2,601 Black participants in the equation's development population, the ethnicity variable was specified as Black or non-Black. The coefficient of 1.159 reflected that the mGFR was 15.9% higher for Black individuals than for non-Black individuals of similar age, sex, and Scr level. It is important to note that race was self-reported and the study population consisted of residents of the United States [53, 62]. In 2021, the Chronic Renal Insufficiency Cohort (CRIC) study showed that regardless of age, sex, and glomerular filtration rate (GFR) measured by $^{125}$I-iothalamate, Black ethnicity was associated with significantly elevated Scr levels. In African Americans, Scr values were 10.7% higher than in individuals of other racial groups. The study also found that for every 10% increase in the percentage of African ancestry determined by genotyping, there was a 1.3% increase in Scr levels [63]. The inclusion of race in the formulation of these equations has recently been debated on the grounds that the inclusion of race in a medical indicator may lead to disparities in access to the health care system, which could manifest as delays in referral to a nephrologist, delays in enrollment in dialysis therapy programs, and waiting lists for kidney transplants. Moreover, as previously mentioned, other important medical decisions are based on eGFR. In 2020, the National Kidney Foundation (NKF) and the American Society of Nephrology formed a Task Force with the goal of reevaluating the scientific evidence that justifies the consideration of ethnicity in the diagnosis and classification of kidney disease [11]. In addition, the Task Force was charged with reviewing the potential clinical impact and diagnostic accuracy that would result from the exclusion of ethnicity in GFR estimation. The aim of this initiative was to bring clarity to this issue and make recommendations that would ensure equitable practice and medical decision-making regardless of the patient's ethnicity. In 2022, the NKF-ASN Task Force recommended that efforts should be made to ensure the accessibility of cystatin C testing for all patients, especially those at risk of CKD [64]. Thus, cystatin C-based equations offer the possibility of estimating GFR and thus defining a medical indicator that supports important medical decisions, regardless of ethnicity, a social and individual condition that goes beyond the biological sphere.

## 6. Estimating glomerular filtration rate (eGFR) by cystatin C in pediatric patients

Due to the significant changes in the child's development, in terms of both maturity and size of the kidneys as well as body growth and muscle mass, challenges arise for each marker of GFR. Although all nephrons are differentiated at birth, only the juxtamedullary glomeruli are immediately utilized, with continuous recruitment of additional glomeruli until the age of 18–24 months. At the age of 2 years, the child has a mGFR-inulin of 105.2 ± 17.3 mL/min/1.73m$^2$ [65] and a mGFR-$^{51}$Cr-EDTA of 104.4 ± 19.9 mL/

min/1.73m$^2$ [66, 67], which is already closer to the GFR of a young adult (on average 120 mL/min/1.73 m$^2$). For comparison purposes for the same child at different stages and in relation to the GFR of an adult, and for the diagnosis and classification of CKD, the value obtained must be expressed in standard units of body surface area. This leads to a close correlation with kidney weight, which would be the ideal reference but is not achievable in practice [68]. Creatinine is the most commonly used marker, but changes in muscle mass with growth affect serum creatinine levels, regardless of the mGFR level. Furthermore, laboratory interference with bilirubin from creatinine measurement assays is important in this population given the prevalence of neonatal jaundice and *in vitro* hemolysis that can occur when small samples are collected. The serum concentration of cystatin C is much higher in premature and newborn infants and gradually decreases until 1 year of age, when it becomes constant [69]. CysC is not influenced by biological variables such as weight and muscle mass, which increase as the child grows. Creatinine behaves similarly in the first months of life, but serum levels gradually increase during childhood and adolescence. In general, equations for estimating GFR in children include adjustments of serum creatinine levels for height as a strategy to capture the gradual changes during childhood and adolescence in the dynamic relationship between height/sCr, muscle mass, sex, age, and mGFR. In the equations that employ both markers, Scr and ScysC, the adjustment of height/Scr is included.

Bokenkamp et al. [52] found a higher correlation coefficient for the 1/ScysC relative to the 1/Scr in a study of 83 children (baseline group) (r 0.88 vs. 0.72; P = 0.001), and in 101 children (application group), ScysC estimated the mRFG of inulin, independent of age, sex, weight, and body composition, in contrast to Scr. In the same study with mGFR inulin, the authors edited the first equation to estimate GFR based on cystatin C. Filler and Lepage [51] developed a formula for eGFRcysC in a population of 536 children who underwent plasma clearance of $^{99}$Tc-DTPA with three samples after a single injection. The resulting bias for eGFRcysC was found to be significantly lower compared to the eGFR-Schwartz-cr formula with a bias of +0.3 and 10.7%, respectively.

It should be noted that since the development of the first equations, further equations have been created. Therefore, caution should be used in comparative analysis because the equations use different exogenous markers for mGFR, different assays for creatinine and cystatin C, and the original equations created prior to 2010 used non-standardized assays for cystatin C. Salvador et al. [70] evaluated the performance of 10 equations based on creatinine, cystatin C, or both in 96 children between 0.25 and 17.5 years of age, with iohexol plasma clearance (mGFR). The eGFR-Schwartz-cr equation showed poor accuracy with a P30 of 53% and a median bias of +15.5 mL/min/1.73 m$^2$ for the entire patient group. This result indicates an overestimation of mGFR. The eGFR-Schwartz-cysC and eGFR-Schwartz-CKiD equations, based on ScysC and ScysC-Scr, respectively, showed the highest accuracy with a P30 of 90% for the total group (n = 96). The eGFR-SchwartzcysC equation showed superior accuracy based on the P30 and P10 metrics, especially in the group with mGFR below 60 mL/min/1.73m$^2$ (P10 44% and P30 85%) and the eGFR-Schwartz-CKiD in the group with mGFR above 60 mL/min/1.73m$^2$ (P10 62% and P30 98%).

## 7. Estimation of glomerular filtration rate (GFR) by cystatin C in the elderly population

It is well documented that GFR decreases by 0.75 to 1 mL/min/1.73 m$^2$/year from the age of 40. However, in the elderly population, Scr level may be normal despite a decrease in mGFR between 45 and 60 mL/min/1.73 m$^2$. This is a critical range of glomerular filtration rate (GFR) for the diagnosis of chronic kidney disease (CKD) and for medical decisions aimed at reducing the risk of disease progression. The main challenge in clinical practice is to find a marker that can differentiate between people with CKD and those without CKD at an early stage of the disease. Creatinine is already known to be an effective marker for late-stage CKD, as numerous studies have shown. Schück et al. [71] conducted a study with a sample of 67 elderly people who had an average urinary inulin clearance of 19.8 mL/min/1.73 m$^2$, indicating advanced CKD. The results showed a strong correlation between the reciprocal values of ScysC comparable to the reciprocal value of Scr when evaluating the AUC-ROC curve and the cutoff of 20 and 10 mL/min/1.73m$^2$ of mGFR-inulin. There was a slight tendency for cystatin C to perform slightly better. Based on the clear knowledge that renal dysfunction is associated with inflammation and higher cardiovascular mortality, CysC can predict cardiovascular risk, perhaps because it is able to distinguish individuals with CKD more quickly. Shlipak et al. [72] published the results of a longitudinal study of 4,637 older participants from the Cardiovascular Healthy Study (CHS) cohort with an average follow-up of 7.4 years. Their analysis showed that the ScysC level was a strong and independent predictor of risk of death and cardiovascular events, outperforming the Scr or eGFRcr-MDRD equation. In another analysis of the same cohort published in 2006 [73], which included older people with an estimated glomerular filtration rate (eGFRcr-MDRD) of ≥60 mL/min/1.73m$^2$, ScysC was found to be significantly correlated with an increased risk of mortality, heart failure, myocardial infarction, and stroke. In contrast, creatinine showed only minimal statistical significance for these correlations. These results suggest that cystatin C may serve as a valuable tool for identifying preclinical renal disease. In addition, eGFRcysC is a reliable indicator of GFR that also has prognostic significance. This is evidenced by the clear and strong association between eGFRcysC and adverse outcomes in individuals aged 60 years and older without a diagnosis of CKD according to the standard criteria of eGFRcr measurements. In a study published in 2023 from the UK Biobank prospective cohort study of 428,402 participants, 76,629 of whom were older, 8% of them had eGFRcysC of less than 60 mL/min/1.73 m$^2$ despite an eGFRcr ≥60 mL/min/1.73 m$^2$, and they had a significantly higher risk of adverse outcomes, suggesting that eGFR-CKDEPIcr overestimates GFR in the absence of eGFRcys measurement and underestimates the risks of CVD and death associated with CKD [74]. An important consideration is the selection of the appropriate equation for the assessment of eGFRcysc in older people. In 2024, the KDIGO update recommended equations developed by CKD-EPI and EKFC, as well as adaptations of these equations that were made in specific regions around the world. CKD-EPI2021 enrolled approximately 695 (13%) participants aged 65 years and older in the equation development dataset. Similar percentages were included in the internal (12%) and external (15%) validation samples [45]. The Berlin Initiative Study (BIS) equation was developed in a study specifically designed for this purpose, which exclusively examined older people aged 70 and over. The study included 610 participants from the BIS cohort (n = 2,073) who had an mGFR based on plasma clearance of iohexol. Two equations were processed: BIS1, based on creatinine, and BIS2, based on cystatin C and creatinine. The lowest bias was found for BIS2 [75]. Fan et al. [76] evaluated the performance of four equations (CKDEPI2012, CAPA, Japanese, and BIS) in a population of 805 elderly individuals with a mean age of 80.3 ± 4.0 years and measured GFR using plasma clearance of iohexol. They found that the combined equation CKDEPIcysC-cr-2012 showed superior performance. In a study of 95 individuals aged 85.3 ± 4.3 years in whom plasma clearance of iohexol was determined, Lopes et al. [77] also observed superior accuracy for the CKDEPIcysC-cr-2012 and BIScysC-cr equations (BIS2). A meta-analysis published in 2023 showed that the combined equations performed better compared to those using an isolated marker [78]. Therefore, in older people, the best method for estimating GFR is the combined eGFRcr-cysC equation.

## 8. Cystatin C in dialysis and kidney transplant patients

In dialysis patients, the measurement of residual kidney function (RKF) is usually determined by the average creatinine and urea clearance. This method is classically recognized in both clinical practice and research, although it has many limitations given the dynamic changes in the interdialytic period, whether due to metabolism, protein intake, or the volume of distribution of these markers, in addition to the difficulties in urine collection. Cystatin C, as well as β2 microglobulin, creatinine, and urea, does not reach stable blood levels in the interdialytic period, limiting the use of these markers as an accurate measure of RKF. Dialysis patients are not represented in the data samples from the development of the currently available eGFR equations. This is a necessary area of research given the known association of RKF with clinical outcomes and patient survival and is also part of the peritoneal dialysis adequacy. Cystatin C is removed during peritoneal dialysis and high-flow hemodialysis and has been studied as a marker of dialysis adequacy in the latter. In kidney transplant patients, validation studies of the current equations for eGFRcr, eGFRcysC, and eGFRcr-cysC show conflicting results, and most studies have samples consisting mainly of White individuals. There is a trend toward using combined equations with cystatin C and creatinine instead of equations based on cystatin C alone. This is an area that requires research with a larger sample of kidney transplant patients to develop and validate an equation, perhaps specifically for use in this population of CKD with a kidney transplant.

## 9. Drug-dosing

Many drugs are excreted by the kidneys *via* glomerular filtration, secretion, metabolism, and tubular reabsorption, so when GFR is reduced, dose adjustment is usually required to prevent or minimize adverse renal and extra-renal effects. Even if the drug is excreted by other routes, the presence of renal insufficiency may affect the volume of distribution and excretion of the drug. For dose adjustment, it is usually recommended to use the non-indexed eGFR, that is, in mL/min and not the eGFR in mL/min/1.73m$^2$, as the renal clearance of a given drug is proportional to the individual's surface GFR. Although the current standard is to use eGFRcr, recent publications have confirmed the accuracy of eGFRcysC without ethnicity factor in predicting target blood level and drug clearance [79–81], data that strongly suggest that cystatin C should also be used for this purpose.

## 10. Conclusion

The glomerular filtration rate (GFR) is the most reliable indicator of kidney function, and its estimation is of paramount importance for many medical decisions.

Equations that estimate eGFR based on cystatin C are accurate and precise in many populations, providing the opportunity to exclude ethnicities from a medical indicator. It is critical to know the non-GFR determinants for each GFR marker to ensure accurate interpretation of results in a variety of clinical scenarios. In this context, the use of equations combined with cystatin C and creatinine shows better performance than equations using isolated markers in children, adults, and the elderly. The current challenge is to disseminate knowledge of cystatin C to physicians and institutional managers in a process of awareness raising to increase demand for the test, thereby reducing costs and facilitating widespread use. The use of cystatin C across the spectrum of renal replacement therapy, including peritoneal dialysis, hemodialysis and its modalities, and kidney transplantation, represents an area of considerable interest that requires new scientific research. Cystatin C-based eGFR has established itself in current clinical practice as a confirmatory test for diagnosis and has important prognostic implications for the most accurate staging of CKD, a growing public health problem worldwide.

## Conflict of interest

The authors declare no conflict of interest.

## Author details

Flávia S. Reis[1*] and Elias David-Neto[2]

1 Faculty of Medicine of Jundiaí, Division of Nephrology, Department of Internal Medicine, Jundiaí, São Paulo, Brazil

2 School of Medicine, Hospital das Clínicas - University of Sao Paulo, Sao Paulo, Brazil

*Address all correspondence to: flaviareis@g.fmj.br

**IntechOpen**

## References

[1] Shannon JA, Smith HW. The excretion of inulin, xylose and urea by normal and phlorizinized man 1. Journal of Clinical Investigation. 1935;**14**(4):393-401

[2] Shannon JA. The renal excretion of creatinine in man. Journal of Clinical Investigation. 1935;**14**(4):403-410

[3] Shemesh O, Golbetz H, Kriss JP, Myers BD. Limitations of creatinine as a filtration marker in glomerulopathic patients. Kidney International. 1985;**28**(5):830-838

[4] Simonsen O, Grubb A, Thysell H. The blood serum concentration of cystatin c (γtrace) as a measure of the glomerular filtration rate. Scandinavian Journal of Clinical and Laboratory Investigation. 1985;**45**(2):97-101

[5] Grubb A, Simonsen O, Sturfelt G, Truedsson L, Thysell H. Serum concentration of cystatin C, factor D and β2-microglobulin as a measure of glomerular filtration rate. Acta Medica Scandinavica. 1985;**218**(5):499-503

[6] Dharnidharka VR, Kwon C, Stevens G. Serum cystatin C is superior to serum creatinine as a marker of kidney function: A meta-analysis. American Journal of Kidney Diseases. 2002;**40**(2):221-226

[7] Levey AS, Coresh J, Bolton K, Culleton B, Harvey KS, Ikizler TA, et al. K/DOQI clinical practice guidelines for chronic kidney disease: Evaluation, classification, and stratification. American Journal of Kidney Diseases. Feb 2002;**39**(2 Suppl 1):1-266

[8] Grubb A, Blirup-Jensen S, Lindström V, Schmidt C, Althaus H, Zegers I. First certified reference material for cystatin C in human serum ERM-DA471/IFCC. Clinical Chemistry and Laboratory Medicine. 2010;**48**(11):1619-1621

[9] Levin A, Stevens PE, Bilous RW, Coresh J, De Francisco ALM, De Jong PE, et al. Kidney Disease: Improving Global Outcomes (KDIGO) CKD Work Group. KDIGO 2012 clinical practice guideline for the evaluation and management of chronic kidney disease. Kidney International Supplements. 2013;**84**(3):622-623

[10] Stevens PE, Ahmed SB, Carrero JJ, Foster B, Francis A, Hall RK, et al. KDIGO 2024 clinical practice guideline for the evaluation and management of chronic kidney disease. Kidney International. 2024;**105**(4S):S117-S314

[11] Delgado C, Baweja M, Burrows NR, Crews DC, Eneanya ND, Gadegbeku CA, et al. Reassessing the inclusion of race in diagnosing kidney diseases: An interim report from the NKF-ASN task force. Journal of the American Society of Nephrology. 2021;**32**(6):1305-1317

[12] Grubb A, Lofberg H, Human γ-trace. Structure, function and clinical use of concentration measurements. Scandinavian Journal of Clinical and Laboratory Investigation. 1985;**45**(Suppl. 177):7-13

[13] Clausen J. Proteins in Normal cerebrospinal fluid not found in serum. Proceedings of the Society for Experimental Biology and Medicine. 1961;**107**(1):170-172

[14] Butler EA, Flynn FV. The occurrence of post-gamma protein in urine: A new

protein abnormality. Journal of Clinical Pathology. 1961;**14**(2):172-178

[15] Jacobsson B, Lignelid H, Bergerheim USR. Transthyretin and cystatin C are catabolized in proximal tubular epithelial cells and the proteins are not useful as markers for renal cell carcinomas. Histopathology. 1995;**26**(6):559-564

[16] Kaseda R, Iino N, Hosojima M, Takeda T, Hosaka K, Kobayashi A, et al. Megalin-mediated endocytosis of cystatin C in proximal tubule cells. Biochemical and Biophysical Research Communications. 2007;**357**(4):1130-1134

[17] Shlipak MG, Mattes MD, Peralta CA. Update on cystatin C: Incorporation into clinical practice. American Journal of Kidney Diseases. 2013;**62**(3):595-603

[18] Knight EL, Verhave JC, Spiegelman D, Hillege HL, De Zeeuw D, Curhan GC, et al. Factors influencing serum cystatin C levels other than renal function and the impact on renal function measurement. Kidney International. 2004;**65**(4):1416-1421

[19] Stevens LA, Schmid CH, Greene T, Li L, Beck GJ, Joffe MM, et al. Factors other than glomerular filtration rate affect serum cystatin C levels. Kidney International. 2009;**75**(6):652-660

[20] Liu X, Foster MC, Tighiouart H, Anderson AH, Beck GJ, Contreras G, et al. Non-GFR determinants of low-molecular-weight serum protein filtration markers in CKD. American Journal of Kidney Diseases. 2016;**68**(6):892-900

[21] Foster MC, Levey AS, Inker LA, Shafi T, Fan L, Gudnason V, et al. Non-GFR determinants of low-molecular-weight serum protein filtration markers in the elderly: AGES-kidney and MESA-kidney. American Journal of Kidney Diseases. 2017;**70**(3):406-414

[22] Schei J, Stefansson VTN, Mathisen UD, Eriksen BO, Solbu MD, Jenssen TG, et al. Residual associations of inflammatory markers with eGFR after accounting for measured GFR in a community-based cohort without CKD. Clinical Journal of the American Society of Nephrology. 2016;**11**(2):280-286

[23] Al-Malki N, Heidenheim PA, Filler G, Yasin A, Lindsay RM. Cystatin C levels in functionally anephric patients undergoing dialysis: The effect of different methods and intensities. Clinical Journal of the American Society of Nephrology. 2009;**4**(10):1606-1610

[24] Okura T, Jotoku M, Irita J, Enomoto D, Nagao T, Desilva VR, et al. Association between cystatin C and inflammation in patients with essential hypertension. Clinical and Experimental Nephrology. 2010;**14**(6):584-588

[25] Grubb A, Björk J, Nyman U, Pollak J, Bengzon J, Östner G, et al. Cystatin C, a marker for successful aging and glomerular filtration rate, is not influenced by inflammation. Scandinavian Journal of Clinical and Laboratory Investigation. 2011;**71**(2):145-149

[26] Muntner P, Winston J, Uribarri J, Mann D, Fox CS. Overweight, obesity, and elevated serum cystatin C levels in adults in the United States. American Journal of Medicine. 2008;**121**(4):341-348

[27] Chew-Harris JSC, Florkowski CM, George PM, Elmslie JL, Endre ZH. The relative effects of fat versus muscle mass on cystatin C and estimates of renal function in healthy young men. Annals of Clinical Biochemistry. 2013;**50**(1):39-46

[28] Naour N, Fellahi S, Renucci JF, Poitou C, Rouault C, Basdevant A, et al. Potential contribution of adipose tissue to elevated serum cystatin C in human obesity. Obesity. 2009;**17**(12):2121-2126

[29] Gruev T, Chakalarovski K, Stojceva-Taneva O, Grueva A, Trenceva K. Effects of glucocorticoid immunosuppression on serum cystatin C levels. Journal of Medical Biochemistry. 2009;**28**(3):191-196

[30] Risch L, Herklotz R, Blumberg A, Huber AR. Effects of glucocorticoid immunosuppression on serum cystatin C concentrations in renal transplant patients. Clinical Chemistry. 2001;**47**(11):2055-2059

[31] Bökenkamp A, Van Wijk JAE, Lentze MJ, Stoffel-Wagner B. Effect of corticosteroid therapy on serum cystatin C and β2-microglobulin concentrations. Clinical Chemistry. 2002;**48**(7):1123-1125

[32] Bjarnadóttir M, Grubb A, Ólafsson Í. Promoter-mediated, dexamethasone-induced increase in cystatin c production by hela cells. Scandinavian Journal of Clinical and Laboratory Investigation. 1995;**55**(7):617-623

[33] Claus T, Elitok S, Schmitt R, Luft FC, Kettritz R. Thyroid function and glomerular filtration - a potential for grave errors. Nephrology Dialysis Transplantation. 2005;**20**(5):1002-1003

[34] Jayagopal V, Keevil BG, Atkin SL, Jennings PE, Kilpatrick ES. Paradoxical changes in cystatin C and serum creatinine in patients with hypo- and hyperthyroidism. Clinical Chemistry. 2003;**49**(4):680-681

[35] Horio M, Imai E, Yasuda Y, Watanabe T, Matsuo S. GFR estimation using standardized serum cystatin C in Japan. American Journal of Kidney Diseases. 2013;**61**(2):197-203

[36] Inker LA, Schmid CH, Tighiouart H, Eckfeldt JH, Feldman HI, Greene T, et al. Estimating glomerular filtration rate from serum creatinine and cystatin C. New England Journal of Medicine. 2012;**367**(1):20-29

[37] Stevens LA, Coresh J, Schmid CH, Feldman HI, Froissart M, Kusek J, et al. Estimating GFR using serum cystatin C alone and in combination with serum creatinine: A pooled analysis of 3,418 individuals with CKD. American Journal of Kidney Diseases. 2008;**51**(3):395-406

[38] Rule AD, Bergstralh EJ, Slezak JM, Bergert J, Larson TS. Glomerular filtration rate estimated by cystatin C among different clinical presentations. Kidney International. 2006;**69**(2):399-405

[39] Hoek FJ, Kemperman FAW, Krediet RT. A comparison between cystatin C, plasma creatinine and the Cockcroft and gault formula for the estimation of glomerular filtration rate. Nephrology Dialysis Transplantation. 2003;**18**(10):2024-2031

[40] Pottel H, Björk J, Rule AD, Ebert N, Eriksen BO, Dubourg L, et al. Cystatin C–based equation to estimate GFR without the inclusion of race and sex. New England Journal of Medicine. 2023;**388**(4):333-343

[41] Pottel H, Delanaye P, Schaeffner E, Dubourg L, Eriksen BO, Melsom T, et al. Estimating glomerular filtration rate for the full age spectrum from serum creatinine and cystatin C. Nephrology Dialysis Transplantation. 2017;**32**(3):497-507

[42] Grubb A, Horio M, Hansson LO, Björk J, Nyman U, Flodin M, et al.

Generation of a new cystatin C-based estimating equation for glomerular filtration rate by use of 7 assays standardized to the international calibrator. Clinical Chemistry. 2014;**60**(7):974-986

[43] Grubb A, Nyman U, Björk J, Lindström V, Rippe B, Sterner G, et al. Simple cystatin C-based prediction equations for glomerular filtration rate compared with the modification of diet in renal disease prediction equation for adults and the Schwartz and the Counahan-Barratt prediction equations for children. Clinical Chemistry. 2005;**51**(8):1420-1431

[44] Larsson A, Malm J, Grubb A, Hansson LO. Calculation of glomerular filtration rate expressed in mL/min from plasma cystatin C values in mg/L. Scandinavian Journal of Clinical and Laboratory Investigation. 2004;**64**(1):25-30

[45] Inker LA, Eneanya ND, Coresh J, Tighiouart H, Wang D, Sang Y, et al. New creatinine- and cystatin C–based equations to estimate GFR without race. New England Journal of Medicine. 2021;**385**(19):1737-1749

[46] Chehade H, Cachat F, Jannot AS, Meyrat BJ, Mosig D, Bardy D, et al. New combined serum creatinine and cystatin C quadratic formula for GFR assessment in children. Clinical Journal of the American Society of Nephrology. 2014;**9**(1):54-63

[47] Schwartz GJ, Schneider MF, Maier PS, Moxey-Mims M, Dharnidharka VR, Warady BA, et al. Improved equations estimating GFR in children with chronic kidney disease using an immunonephelometric determination of cystatin C. Kidney International. 2012;**82**(4):445-453

[48] Schwartz GJ, Muñoz A, Schneider MF, Mak RH, Kaskel F, Warady BA, et al. New equations to estimate GFR in children with CKD. Journal of the American Society of Nephrology. 2009;**20**(3):629-637

[49] Zappitelli M, Parvex P, Joseph L, Paradis G, Grey V, Lau S, et al. Derivation and validation of cystatin C-based prediction equations for GFR in children. American Journal of Kidney Diseases. 2006;**48**(2):221-230

[50] Pierce CB, Muñoz A, Ng DK, Warady BA, Furth SL, Schwartz GJ. Age and sex-dependent clinical equations to estimate glomerular filtration rates in children and young adults with chronic kidney disease. Kidney International. 2021;**99**(4):948-956

[51] Filler G, Lepage N. Should the Schwartz formula for estimation of GFR be replaced by cystatin C formula? Pediatric Nephrology. 2003;**18**(10):981-985

[52] Bökenkamp A, Domanetzki M, Zinck R, Schumann G, Byrd D, Brodehl J. Cystatin C - A new marker of glomerular filtration rate in children independent of age and height. Pediatrics. 1998;**101**(5):875-881

[53] Levey AS, Stevens LA, Schmid CH, Zhang Y, Castro AF, Feldman HI, et al. A new equation to estimate glomerular filtration rate. Annals of Internal Medicine. 2009;**150**(9):604-612

[54] Pottel H, Björk J, Courbebaisse M, Couzi L, Ebert N, Eriksen BO, et al. Development and validation of a modified full age spectrum creatinine-based equation to estimate glomerular filtration rate. Annals of Internal Medicine. 2021;**174**(2):183-191

[55] Shlipak MG, Matsushita K, Ärnlöv J, Inker LA, Katz R, Polkinghorne KR,

et al. Cystatin C versus creatinine in determining risk based on kidney function. New England Journal of Medicine. 2013;**369**(10):932-943

[56] Peralta CA, Shlipak MG, Judd S, Cushman M, McClellan W, Zakai NA, et al. Detection of chronic kidney disease with creatinine, cystatin c, and urine albumin-to-creatinine ratio and association with progression to end-stage renal disease and mortality. Journal of the American Medical Association. 2011;**305**(15):1545-1552

[57] Chen DC, Shlipak MG, Scherzer R, Bauer SR, Potok OA, Rifkin DE, et al. Association of intraindividual difference in estimated glomerular filtration rate by creatinine vs cystatin C and end-stage kidney disease and mortality. JAMA Network Open. 2022;**5**(2):1-14

[58] Adingwupu OM, Barbosa ER, Palevsky PM, Vassalotti JA, Levey AS, Inker LA. Cystatin C as a GFR estimation marker in acute and chronic illness: A systematic review. Kidney Medicine. 2023;**5**(12):1-14

[59] Fu EL, Levey AS, Coresh J, Grams ME, Faucon AL, Elinder CG, et al. Accuracy of GFR estimating equations based on creatinine, cystatin C or both in routine care. Nephrology Dialysis Transplantation. 2024;**39**(4):694-706

[60] Pottel H, Hoste L, Dubourg L, Ebert N, Schaeffner E, Eriksen BO, et al. An estimated glomerular filtration rate equation for the full age spectrum. Nephrology Dialysis Transplantation. 2016;**31**(5):798-806

[61] Teo BW, Zhang L, Guh JY, Tang SCW, Jha V, Kang DH, et al. Glomerular filtration rates in Asians. Advances in Chronic Kidney Disease. 2018;**25**(1): 41-48

[62] Levey AS, Titan SM, Powe NR, Coresh J, Inker LA. Kidney disease, race, and GFR estimation. Clinical Journal of the American Society of Nephrology. 2020;**15**(8):1203-1212

[63] Hsu C, Yang W, Parikh RV, Anderson AH, Chen TK, Cohen DL, et al. Race, genetic ancestry, and estimating kidney function in CKD. New England Journal of Medicine. 2021;**385**(19):1750-1760

[64] Delgado C, Baweja M, Crews DC, Eneanya ND, Gadegbeku CA, Inker LA, et al. A unifying approach for GFR estimation: Recommendations of the NKF-ASN task force on reassessing the inclusion of race in diagnosing kidney disease. American Journal of Kidney Diseases. 2022;**79**(2):268-288

[65] Schwartz GJ, Furth SL. Glomerular filtration rate measurement and estimation in chronic kidney disease. Pediatric Nephrology. 2007;**22**(11):1839-1848

[66] Piepsz A, Tondeur M, Ham H. Revisiting normal $^{51}$Cr-ethylenediaminetetraacetic acid clearance values in children. European Journal of Nuclear Medicine and Molecular Imaging. 2006;**33**(12):1477-1482

[67] Jančič SG, Močnik M, Marčun VN. Glomerular filtration rate assessment in children. Children. 2022;**9**:1-12

[68] Filler G, Yasin A, Medeiros M. Methods of assessing renal function. Pediatric Nephrology. 2014;**29**(2):183-192

[69] Bökenkamp A, Domanetzki M, Zinck R, Schumann G, Brodehl J. Reference values for cystatin C serum concentrations in children. Pediatric Nephrology. 1998;**12**(2):125-129

[70] Salvador CL, Tøndel C, Rowe AD, Bjerre A, Brun A, Brackman D, et al. Estimating glomerular filtration rate in children: Evaluation of creatinine- and cystatin C-based equations. Pediatric Nephrology. 2019;**34**(2):301-311

[71] Schück O, Teplan V, Jabor A, Stollova M, Skibova J. Glomerular filtration rate estimation in patients with advanced chronic renal insufficiency based on serum cystatin C levels. Nephron. Clinical Practice. 2003;**93**(4):c146-c151

[72] Shlipak MG, Sarnak MJ, Katz R, Fried LF, Seliger SL, Newman AB, et al. Cystatin C and the risk of death and cardiovascular events among elderly persons. New England Journal of Medicine. 2005;**352**(20):2049-2060

[73] Shlipak MG, Katz R, Sarnak MJ, Fried LF, Newman AB, Stehman-Breen C, et al. Cystatin C and prognosis for cardiovascular and kidney outcomes in elderly persons without chronic kidney disease. Annals of Internal Medicine. 2006;**145**(4):237-246

[74] Lees JS, Rutherford E, Stevens KI, Chen DC, Scherzer R, Estrella MM, et al. Assessment of cystatin C level for risk stratification in adults with chronic kidney disease. JAMA Network Open. 2022;**5**(10):1-14

[75] Schaeffner ES, Ebert N, Delanaye P, Frei U, Gaedeke J, Jakob O, et al. Two novel equations to estimate kidney function in persons aged 70 years or older. Annals of Internal Medicine. 2012;**157**(7):471-481

[76] Fan L, Levey AS, Gudnason V, Eiriksdottir G, Andresdottir MB, Gudmundsdottir H, et al. Comparing GFR estimating equations using cystatin C and creatinine in elderly individuals.

Journal of the American Society of Nephrology. 2015;**26**(8):1982-1989

[77] Lopes MB, Araújo LQ, Passos MT, Nishida SK, Kirsztajn GM, Cendoroglo MS, et al. Estimation of glomerular filtration rate from serum creatinine and cystatin C in octogenarians and nonagenarians. BMC Nephrology. 2013;**14**(1):1-9

[78] Ma Y, Shen X, Yong Z, Wei L, Zhao W. Comparison of glomerular filtration rate estimating equations in older adults: A systematic review and meta-analysis. Archives of Gerontology and Geriatrics. 2023;**114**:1-8

[79] Barreto EF, Rule AD, Murad MH, Kashani KB, Lieske JC, Erwin PJ, et al. Prediction of the renal elimination of drugs with cystatin C vs creatinine: A systematic review. Mayo Clinic Proceedings. 2019;**94**(3):500-514

[80] Yu G, Li GF. Is cystatin C good enough as a biomarker for vancomycin dosing: A pharmacokinetic perspective. European Journal of Drug Metabolism and Pharmacokinetics. 2020;**45**(1):151-156

[81] Yun HG, Smith AJF, DeBacker KC, Pai MP. Estimated glomerular filtration rate with and without race for drug dosing: Cystatin C vs. serum creatinine. British Journal of Clinical Pharmacology. 2023;**89**(3):1207-1210

# Perspective Chapter: Big Data and Artificial Intelligence in Cystatin C Research

*Smita Kumbhar and Manish Bhatia*

## Abstract

This chapter explores the integration of Big Data and Artificial Intelligence (AI) in the context of Cystatin C research—a pivotal biomarker for assessing renal function, cardiovascular health, and certain neurodegenerative conditions. It begins by establishing the clinical relevance of Cystatin C and its advantages over conventional biomarkers such as creatinine. The discussion then shifts to the role of Big Data, encompassing diverse sources like electronic health records, genomic datasets, medical imaging, and data from wearable devices. These multimodal data streams provide a holistic framework for understanding Cystatin C's role in disease prediction and management. Key challenges such as data heterogeneity, privacy concerns, and interoperability issues are highlighted. The chapter further illustrates the application of AI methods—including machine learning, deep learning, and natural language processing—in processing complex datasets to enhance diagnostic precision, forecast disease progression, and inform individualized treatment strategies. Several case studies underscore the practical utility of these approaches, particularly in chronic kidney disease monitoring, cardiovascular risk prediction, and early detection of neurological decline. Looking ahead, the chapter advocates for deeper integration of predictive analytics, refinement of computational models, and ethical frameworks to guide AI deployment. It concludes that leveraging Big Data and AI in Cystatin C research presents significant opportunities to improve the clinical outcomes and catalyze innovation in diagnostics and therapeutics. Continued interdisciplinary collaboration among clinicians, data scientists, and researchers will be critical to realizing this potential.

**Keywords:** cystatin C, big data, artificial intelligence, machine learning, deep learning, biomarkers

## 1. Introduction

The integration of Big Data and Artificial Intelligence (AI) into biomedical research has significantly reshaped clinical diagnostics and therapeutic strategies, offering unprecedented insights into complex disease mechanisms. Among emerging biomarkers, Cystatin C has garnered attention as a superior marker of glomerular filtration rate (GFR), with broader implications in cardiovascular, metabolic, and neurodegenerative diseases [1, 2]. Unlike traditional markers such as serum creatinine, Cystatin C demonstrates greater stability across age, sex, and muscle mass variations [3, 4]. This chapter explores how Big Data and AI synergistically enhance the study and clinical utility of Cystatin C, transforming it from a standalone marker to a predictive tool within the integrated health ecosystems.

## 1.1 The role of cystatin C in medical research

Cystatin C is a non-glycosylated, 13-kDa protein from the cystatin superfamily, constitutively expressed by all nucleated cells and rapidly cleared *via* renal filtration [3]. Because it is neither secreted by renal tubules nor significantly influenced by extrarenal factors, its serum levels provide a highly sensitive estimate of kidney function [4]. Multiple studies have demonstrated Cystatin C's predictive value in chronic kidney disease (CKD) [5], heart failure and coronary artery disease [6], neurodegenerative conditions such as Alzheimer's disease (AD) and Parkinson's disease (PD) [7], as well as metabolic syndromes and frailty [8]. Moreover, its elevation correlates independently with all-cause mortality in several population-based cohorts [9].

## 1.2 Big data in cystatin C research

### 1.2.1 Definition and importance of big data

Big Data in healthcare comprises voluminous, heterogeneous datasets generated at high speed from disparate sources, including electronic health records (EHRs), genomics, medical imaging, and wearable health devices. Governed by the "4 V's"—Volume, Variety, Velocity, and Veracity—these data offer granular, real-time insights into disease trajectories and treatment outcomes [10]. Within Cystatin C research, these diverse datasets support multifactorial analyses by correlating biochemical levels with phenotypic, genetic, and lifestyle variables.

The integration of Big Data and Artificial Intelligence into Cystatin C research involves a multi-step process encompassing data acquisition, preprocessing, model development, and clinical application (**Figure 1**). This pipeline ensures a structured approach to harness the full potential of diverse data sources and AI methodologies in biomarker analysis.

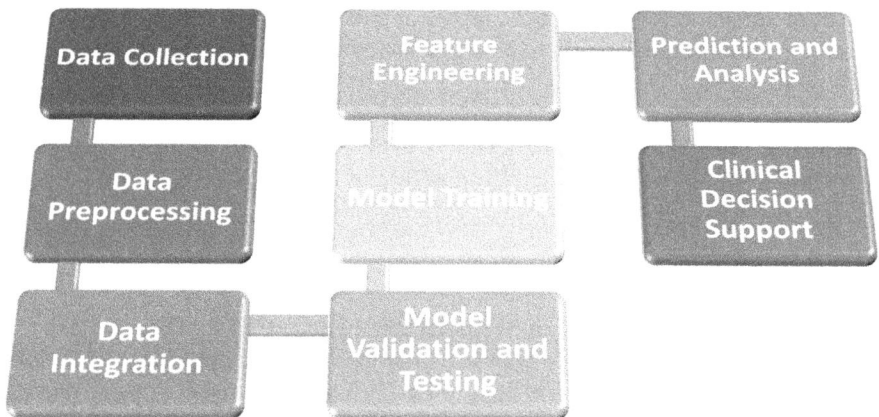

**Figure 1.**
*Flowchart of integration of big data and artificial intelligence in cystatin C research.*

## 1.3 Data sources and types

A wide range of data sources inform the study of Cystatin C. These sources vary in temporal resolution, data richness, and clinical applicability, as shown in **Table 1**.

## 1.4 Challenges in big data integration

Despite its promise, Big Data integration in Cystatin C research faces critical challenges in quality control, privacy, and interoperability. These are summarized in **Table 2**.

## 1.5 Artificial intelligence in cystatin C research

### 1.5.1 Overview of AI technologies

AI, encompassing machine learning (ML), deep learning (DL), and natural language processing (NLP), enables the interpretation of complex, high-dimensional data to uncover hidden patterns and derive actionable insights. These approaches augment traditional clinical analytics, driving precision in disease classification, prognostication, and treatment [18, 19].

### 1.5.2 Machine learning applications

ML algorithms are particularly powerful in risk stratification and predictive analytics involving Cystatin C. These applications are detailed in **Table 3**.

| Data source | Description | Contribution to cystatin C research |
|---|---|---|
| Electronic health records (EHRs) | Lab results, treatment histories, diagnoses | Enables longitudinal tracking and predictive modeling [11] |
| Genomic data | Whole genome/exome sequences, SNP arrays | Links gene polymorphisms to Cystatin C variations [12] |
| Imaging data | MRI, CT, PET, ultrasound scans | Correlates structural changes with Cystatin C levels [13] |
| Wearable devices | Smartwatches, biosensors | Real-time monitoring and behavioral data integration [14] |

**Table 1.**
*Data sources and their contributions to cystatin C research.*

| Challenge | Description | Possible solutions |
|---|---|---|
| Data quality and standardization | Variability in acquisition and format | Unified data schemas, ontologies, validation pipelines [15] |
| Data privacy and security | Exposure of sensitive health information | Encryption, access control, HIPAA/GDPR compliance [16] |
| Interoperability | Platform-specific data silos | Use of FHIR, open APIs, and federated learning [17] |

**Table 2.**
*Challenges in big data integration for cystatin C research.*

| Application | Description | Benefits |
|---|---|---|
| Predictive analytics | Disease trajectory modeling | Early detection of CKD, hospitalization risk [20] |
| Personalized medicine | AI-driven treatment stratification | Customization based on genetic/clinical profiles [21] |
| Disease classification | Multivariate disease subtype recognition | More accurate diagnoses of CKD, CVD, AD [22] |

**Table 3.**
*Machine learning applications in cystatin C research.*

## 1.6 Natural language processing (NLP)

NLP enables the mining of unstructured data, including clinical notes, discharge summaries, and research papers. It has been used to extract Cystatin C trends, co-morbidity patterns, and treatment pathways from large EHR corpora and literature repositories [23].

### 1.6.1 Deep learning applications

Deep learning methods such as convolutional neural networks (CNNs) and recurrent neural networks (RNNs) allow the integration of imaging data and omics layers for advanced diagnostics. For instance, models integrating MRI scans with serum Cystatin C data have demonstrated a > 20% increase in early detection sensitivity for neurodegenerative diseases [24, 25].

### 1.6.2 Case studies and applications

Multiple clinical studies have validated AI models using Cystatin C across diverse domains, as shown in **Table 4**.

## 1.7 Literature review and broader context

Numerous studies illustrate AI's utility in other biomarker domains, offering models for Cystatin C research:

- In cardiac diagnostics, ML has improved prediction using troponin and BNP [29].

- AI-assisted cancer biomarker analysis (e.g., PSA, CA-125) has enhanced early detection and treatment personalization [30].

| Case study | Description | Outcomes and impact |
|---|---|---|
| Predicting chronic kidney disease | ML model using EHR and Cystatin C trajectories | 89% accuracy in early CKD risk identification [26] |
| Cardiovascular risk stratification | AI integration of Cystatin C, genomics, lifestyle | Personalized intervention plans and improved outcomes [27] |
| Neurodegenerative disease classification | DL models on imaging + Cystatin C data | High sensitivity and prognostic utility for AD/PD [28] |

**Table 4.**
*Case studies demonstrating AI applications in cystatin C research.*

- In diabetes, real-time glucose monitoring *via* AI has improved glycemic control [31, 32].

- Alzheimer's diagnostics using CSF proteins and MRI have benefitted from deep learning algorithms [33].

These precedents affirm the translational potential of AI methodologies in optimizing Cystatin C utilization.

## 1.8 Future directions and opportunities

1. Precision medicine: Deep phenotyping *via* AI will allow N-of-1 treatment modeling based on dynamic Cystatin C profiles [34].

2. Multi-omics integration: AI can unify transcriptomic, proteomic, and metabolomic data to elucidate Cystatin C regulation networks [35].

3. Real-time monitoring: Integration of wearable biosensors with mobile health platforms for continuous risk stratification [36].

4. AI Ethics and Fairness: Development of explainable AI (XAI) systems and transparency in Cystatin C predictive tools [37].

5. Telemedicine expansion: Remote diagnostics using AI-integrated devices will support decentralized Cystatin C monitoring [38].

## 2. Conclusion

The convergence of Big Data and AI marks a transformative era in Cystatin C research and clinical application. These technologies enable early diagnosis, real-time monitoring, and individualized care strategies that outperform the traditional models. However, ethical deployment, clinical validation, and interdisciplinary synergy remain essential. As innovation progresses, AI-augmented Cystatin C diagnostics may become integral to global precision medicine frameworks.

## Conflict of interest

The authors declare no conflict of interest.

## Author details

Smita Kumbhar[1*] and Manish Bhatia[2]

1 Department of Pharmaceutical Chemistry, Sanjivani College of Pharmaceutical Education and Research (Autonomous), Kopargaon, Maharashtra, India

2 Department of Pharmaceutical Chemistry, Bharati Vidyapeeth College of Pharmacy, Kolhapur, India

*Address all correspondence to: smitakumbharresearch@gmail.com

**IntechOpen**

# References

[1] Ding L, Liu Z, Wang J. Role of cystatin C in urogenital malignancy. Frontiers in Endocrinology. 2022;**13**:1082871. DOI: 10.3389/fendo.2022.1082871

[2] Leto G, Crescimanno M, Flandina C. On the role of cystatin C in cancer progression. Life Sciences. 2018;**202**:152-160. DOI: 10.1016/j.lfs.2018.04.013

[3] Leto G, Sepporta MV. The potential of cystatin C as a predictive biomarker in breast cancer. Expert Review of Anticancer Therapy. 2020;**20**(12):1049-1056. DOI: 10.1080/14737140.2020.1829481

[4] Nian W, Tao W, Zhang H. Review of research progress in sepsis-associated acute kidney injury. Frontiers in Molecular Biosciences. 2025;**12**:1603392. DOI: 10.3389/fmolb.2025.1603392

[5] Olsson SL, Ek B, Björk I. The affinity and kinetics of inhibition of cysteine proteinases by intact recombinant bovine cystatin C. Biochimica et Biophysica Acta. 1999;**1432**(1):73-81. DOI: 10.1016/s0167-4838(99)00090-4

[6] van Wyk SG, Kunert KJ, Cullis CA, Pillay P, Makgopa ME, Schlüter U, et al. Review: The future of cystatin engineering. Plant Science: An International Journal of Experimental Plant Biology. 2016;**246**:119-127. DOI: 10.1016/j.plantsci.2016.02.016

[7] Amin F, Khan MS, Bano B. Mammalian cystatin and protagonists in brain diseases. Journal of Biomolecular Structure and Dynamics. 2020;**38**(7):2171-2196. DOI: 10.1080/07391102.2019.1620636

[8] Mathews PM, Levy E. Cystatin C in aging and in Alzheimer's disease.

Ageing Research Reviews. 2016;**32**:38-50. DOI: 10.1016/j.arr.2016.06.003

[9] Gauthier S, Kaur G, Mi W, Tizon B, Levy E. Protective mechanisms by cystatin C in neurodegenerative diseases. Frontiers in Bioscience (Scholar Edition). 2011;**3**(2):541-554. DOI: 10.2741/s170

[10] Watanabe S, Hayakawa T, Wakasugi K, Yamanaka K. Cystatin C protects neuronal cells against mutant copper-zinc superoxide dismutase-mediated toxicity. Cell Death and Disease. 2014;**5**(10):e1497. DOI: 10.1038/cddis.2014.459

[11] Tizon B, Sahoo S, Yu H, Gauthier S, Kumar AR, Mohan P, et al. Induction of autophagy by cystatin C: A mechanism that protects murine primary cortical neurons and neuronal cell lines. PLoS One. 2010;**5**(3):e9819. DOI: 10.1371/journal.pone.0009819

[12] Inker LA, Eneanya ND, Coresh J, Tighiouart H, Wang D, Sang Y, et al. New creatinine- and cystatin C-based equations to estimate GFR without race. The New England Journal of Medicine. 2021;**385**(19):1737-1749. DOI: 10.1056/NEJMoa2102953

[13] Luo J, Wang LP, Hu HF, Zhang L, Li YL, Ai LM, et al. Cystatin C and cardiovascular or all-cause mortality risk in the general population: A meta-analysis. Clinica Chimica Acta; International Journal of Clinical Chemistry. 2015;**450**:39-45. DOI: 10.1016/j.cca.2015.07.016

[14] Lind M, Jansson JH, Nilsson TK, Järvholm LS, Johansson L. Cystatin C and creatinine as markers of bleeding complications, cardiovascular events and mortality during oral anticoagulant

treatment. Thrombosis Research. 2013;**132**(2):e77-e82. DOI: 10.1016/j. thromres.2013.06.011

[15] Yang S, Song L, Zhao L, Dong P, Lai L, Wang H. Predictive value of cystatin C in people with suspected or established coronary artery disease: A meta-analysis. Atherosclerosis. 2017;**263**:60-67. DOI: 10.1016/j. atherosclerosis.2017.05.025

[16] Jin S, Xu J, Shen G, Gu P. Predictive value of circulating cystatin C level in patients with acute coronary syndrome: A meta-analysis. Scandinavian Journal of Clinical and Laboratory Investigation. 2021;**81**(1):1-7. DOI: 10.1080/00365513.2020.1846212

[17] Pruc M, Swieczkowski D, Cander B, Jaguszewski MJ, Galwankar S, Di Somma S, et al. Diagnostic and prognostic value of cystatin C in acute coronary syndrome: An up-to-date meta-analysis. Cardiology Journal. 2025;**32**(2):142-152. DOI: 10.5603/cj.102453

[18] Teaford HR, Barreto JN, Vollmer KJ, Rule AD, Barreto EF. Cystatin C: A primer for pharmacists. Pharmacy (Basel, Switzerland). 2020;**8**(1):35. DOI: 10.3390/pharmacy8010035

[19] Laterza OF, Price CP, Scott MG. Cystatin C: An improved estimator of glomerular filtration rate? Clinical Chemistry. 2002;**48**(5):699-707

[20] Narvaez-Sanchez R, Gonzalez L, Salamanca A, Silva M, Rios D, Arevalo S, et al. Cystatin C could be a replacement to serum creatinine for diagnosing and monitoring kidney function in children. Clinical Biochemistry. 2008;**41**(7-8):498-503. DOI: 10.1016/j. clinbiochem.2008.01.022

[21] Sato H, Kuroda T, Tanabe N, Ajiro J, Wada Y, Murakami S, et al. Cystatin C is a sensitive marker for detecting a reduced glomerular filtration rate when assessing chronic kidney disease in patients with rheumatoid arthritis and secondary amyloidosis. Scandinavian Journal of Rheumatology. 2010;**39**(1):33-37. DOI: 10.3109/03009740903042402

[22] Theodorakakou F, Fotiou D, Apostolakou F, Papassotiriou I, Spiliopoulou V, Ntanasis-Stathopoulos I, et al. Cystatin C as biomarker for the evaluation of renal outcome in AL amyloidosis. American Journal of Hematology. 2025;**100**(8):1305-1313. DOI: 10.1002/ajh.27716

[23] Agana BA, Ness MA, Frazier J, Marzinke MA. Evaluation of cystatin C utilization and its discordance with creatinine in a large academic medical center. Clinica Chimica Acta; International Journal of Clinical Chemistry. 2025;**577**:120450. DOI: 10.1016/j.cca.2025.120450

[24] Karger AB, Shlipak MG. Glomerular filtration rate (GFR) estimation with cystatin C-past, present, and future. Clinical Chemistry. 2025;**71**(7):743-751. DOI: 10.1093/clinchem/hvac226

[25] Pottel H, Björk J, Rule AD, Ebert N, Eriksen BO, Dubourg L, et al. Cystatin C-based equation to estimate GFR without the inclusion of race and sex. The New England Journal of Medicine. 2023;**388**(4):333-343. DOI: 10.1056/ NEJMoa2203769

[26] Lafarge JC, Naour N, Clément K, Guerre-Millo M. Cathepsins and cystatin C in atherosclerosis and obesity. Biochimie. 2010;**92**(11):1580-1586. DOI: 10.1016/j.biochi.2010.04.011

[27] Taleb S, Lacasa D, Bastard JP, Poitou C, Cancello R, Pelloux V, et al. Cathepsin S, a novel biomarker of adiposity: Relevance to atherogenesis.

FASEB Journal: Official Publication of the Federation of American Societies for Experimental Biology. 2005;**19**(11):1540-1542. DOI: 10.1096/fj.05-3673fje

[28] Jiang Y, Zhang J, Zhang C, Hong L, Jiang Y, Lu L, et al. The role of cystatin C as a proteasome inhibitor in multiple myeloma. Hematology (Amsterdam, Netherlands). 2020;**25**(1):457-463. DOI: 10.1080/16078454.2020.1850973

[29] Groothof D, Shehab NBN, Erler NS, Post A, Kremer D, Polinder-Bos HA, et al. Creatinine, cystatin C, muscle mass, and mortality: Findings from a primary and replication population-based cohort. Journal of Cachexia, Sarcopenia and Muscle. 2024;**15**(4):1528-1538. DOI: 10.1002/jcsm.13511

[30] He D, Gao B, Wang J, Yang C, Zhao MH, Zhang L. The difference between cystatin C- and creatinine-based estimated glomerular filtration rate and risk of diabetic microvascular complications among adults with diabetes: A population-based cohort study. Diabetes Care. 2024;**47**(5):873-880. DOI: 10.2337/dc23-2364

[31] Fu EL, Levey AS, Coresh J, Grams ME, Faucon AL, Elinder CG, et al. Accuracy of GFR estimating equations based on creatinine, cystatin C or both in routine care. Nephrology, Dialysis, Transplantation: Official Publication of the European Dialysis and Transplant Association - European Renal Association. 2024;**39**(4):694-706. DOI: 10.1093/ndt/gfad219

[32] Visinescu AM, Rusu E, Cosoreanu A, Radulian G. CYSTATIN C-A monitoring perspective of chronic kidney disease in patients with diabetes. International Journal of Molecular Sciences. 2024;**25**(15):8135. DOI: 10.3390/ijms25158135

[33] Skidmore M, Spencer S, Desborough R, Kent D, Bhandari S. Cystatin C as a marker of kidney function in children. Biomolecules. 2024;**14**(8):938. DOI: 10.3390/biom14080938

[34] Kaur G, Levy E. Cystatin C in Alzheimer's disease. Frontiers in Molecular Neuroscience. 2012;**5**:79. DOI: 10.3389/fnmol.2012.00079

[35] Zhang Y, Sun L. Cystatin C in cerebrovascular disorders. Current Neurovascular Research. 2017;**14**(4):406-414. DOI: 10.2174/1567202614666171116102504

[36] Tizon B, Ribe EM, Mi W, Troy CM, Levy E. Cystatin C protects neuronal cells from amyloid-beta-induced toxicity. Journal of Alzheimer's Disease: JAD. 2010;**19**(3):885-894. DOI: 10.3233/JAD-2010-1291

[37] Perlenfein TJ, Murphy RM. A mechanistic model to predict effects of cathepsin B and cystatin C on β-amyloid aggregation and degradation. The Journal of Biological Chemistry. 2017;**292**(51):21071-21082. DOI: 10.1074/jbc.M117.811448

[38] Sun B, Zhou Y, Halabisky B, Lo I, Cho SH, Mueller-Steiner S, et al. Cystatin C-cathepsin B axis regulates amyloid beta levels and associated neuronal deficits in an animal model of Alzheimer's disease. Neuron. 2008;**60**(2):247-257. DOI: 10.1016/j.neuron.2008.10.001

Chapter 4

# The Way of the PCNL

*Alessandro Calarco and Pietro Viscuso*

## Abstract

*"We see what we know, and if we know it, we do not fear it."* This principle, valid across all surgical disciplines, is perhaps even more relevant in percutaneous nephrolithotripsy (PCNL). In particular, the puncture phase relies on anatomical landmarks rather than direct visualization. If we do not learn to "see," we will inevitably fear the procedure. PCNL is performed by a limited number of surgeons, often with varying outcomes and complications. While these complications are frequently dismissed as inevitable, in reality, they almost always stem from technical errors rather than mere chance. We will focus on thoroughly understanding the fundamentals of PCNL, including surgical methodology, technical execution, and strategic approach, explaining the rationale behind every step of the procedure. The goal is to condense everything one needs to master the fundamentals of PCNL into no more than 20 pages while adhering to the first principle of Hippocrates: *"Primum non nocere"* ("First, do no harm"). Do not perform a PCNL if you are not capable. Do not attempt a PCNL without first reading this chapter. Follow the principles outlined here, and you will become a *PercMaster*.

**Keywords:** PCNL, technique, endourology, PercMaster, stones

## 1. Introduction

Percutaneous nephrolithotomy (PCNL) has revolutionized the management of large and complex renal calculi, emerging as a minimally invasive alternative to open stone surgery. The origins of PCNL can be traced back to 1976, when Fernström and Johansson in Sweden performed the first successful procedure by creating a percutaneous tract into the renal pelvis for direct stone extraction. This groundbreaking approach laid the foundation for the development of dedicated instruments and techniques that would shape modern urology.

In its earliest days, PCNL relied on modified endoscopic tools originally designed for other surgical applications. Rigid nephroscopes and basic dilators were adapted to create and maintain the percutaneous access tract. The introduction of ultrasonic and electrohydraulic lithotripters in the late 1970s and early 1980s significantly improved the ability to fragment and extract stones, reducing operative times and complications. The 1980s also saw the advent of balloon dilators and Amplatz sheath systems, which standardized tract creation and minimized trauma to the renal parenchyma.

A major leap occurred in the 1990s with the miniaturization of instruments, leading to the development of mini-PCNL techniques. Advances in fiber optics and the introduction of flexible nephroscopes allowed for enhanced visualization and access to complex intrarenal anatomy. Meanwhile, improvements in energy sources, including the advent of holmium:YAG lasers, provided more effective and versatile options for intracorporeal lithotripsy.

In the twenty-first century, further innovations such as micro-PCNL, ultra-mini PCNL, and disposable instruments have aimed to reduce morbidity and simplify the procedure. Advances in imaging modalities, including real-time fluoroscopy, ultrasound-guided access, and even robotic assistance, have further refined the precision and safety of PCNL. Today, the procedure continues to evolve, driven by ongoing innovation in instrumentation and technology, cementing its role as the gold standard for treating complex renal stones.

## 2. Ensuring success: Surgical proficiency and team coordination in PCNL

The success of percutaneous nephrolithotomy (PCNL) relies heavily on a thorough understanding of the procedural steps and meticulous execution by the surgical team. While PCNL is considered a minimally invasive procedure, its complexity demands precise planning and technical expertise to minimize risks and optimize outcomes. A well-prepared surgical team plays a pivotal role in achieving this goal, as familiarity with the instruments, surgical workflow, and intraoperative challenges is essential for seamless coordination. From obtaining accurate percutaneous access to managing potential complications, the collaborative effort of the surgeon, anesthesiologist, and operating room staff ensures procedural efficiency and patient safety. By mastering each step of the procedure and fostering a culture of teamwork, PCNL can be performed effectively and with a high degree of reproducibility, making it an accessible and successful intervention in the management of renal stones.

According to the guidelines of the *European Association of Urology (EAU)* and the *American Urological Association (AUA)*, preoperative imaging for PCNL is essential for accurate surgical planning and reducing the risk of complications [1, 2].

The primary recommendations include:

- *Non-contrast computed tomography (CT)*: considered the first-choice examination, providing precise details on the size, location, and composition of stones, as well as essential anatomical information of the urinary system.

- *Magnetic resonance imaging (MRI)*: though less common, it can be considered in patients with contraindications to CT or ionizing radiation.

- *Ultrasound*: useful as a complementary tool to evaluate hydronephrosis and guide percutaneous access, but with limitations in detecting small or radiolucent stones.

Additionally, assessing renal function through preoperative laboratory tests is essential, and the use of contrast agents should be considered based on the patient's renal functionality, following guidelines on contrast agent safety.

In summary, a comprehensive preoperative evaluation through imaging is crucial for the success of PCNL, and the choice of diagnostic modalities should be tailored based on the patient's clinical conditions and available resources (**Figure 1**).

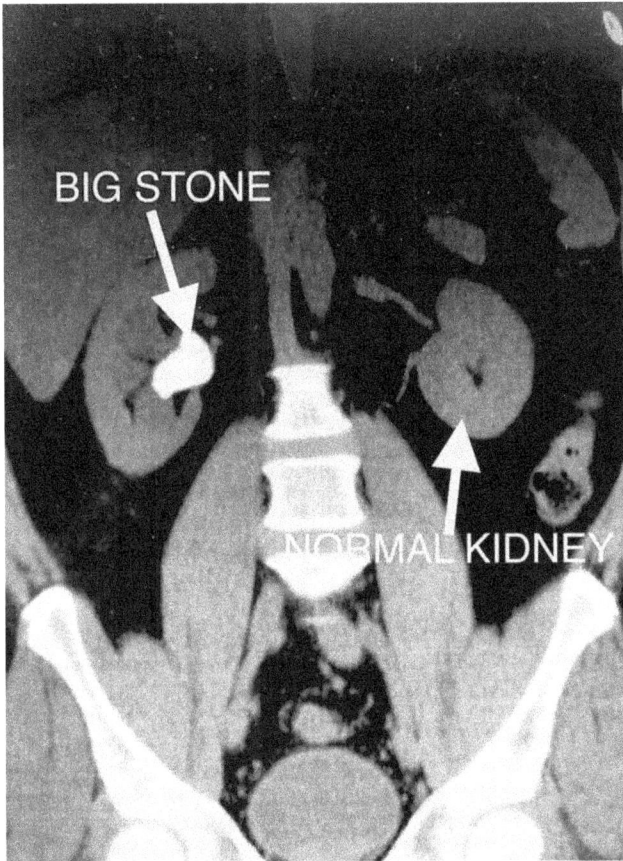

**Figure 1.**
*Comparison between a normal kidney and a kidney with stone.*

## 3. Indications for PCNL

Percutaneous nephrolithotomy (PCNL) is the first-line treatment for patients with large, complex, or symptomatic renal stones, as outlined by both the AUA and EAU guidelines. The procedure is indicated in cases where the size, composition, or anatomical location of the stones render less invasive modalities, such as extracorporeal shock wave lithotripsy (ESWL) or ureteroscopy (URS), less effective or impractical. Several validated scoring systems are available to assist surgeons in the decision-making process [3–5].

According to the AUA and EAU, specific indications for PCNL include (**Table 1**).

1. *Large stone burden*: Stones >20 mm in diameter are the primary indication for PCNL, as the procedure achieves higher stone-free rates compared to ESWL or URS.

2. *Staghorn calculi*: PCNL is the standard treatment for staghorn stones, which involve the renal pelvis and calyces, due to its ability to address extensive stone burden effectively.

| Indication | Details | Alternative Treatment |
|---|---|---|
| Stone size >20 mm | Higher stone-free rates for large stones. | ESWL (limited efficacy for large stones). |
| Staghorn calculi | Gold standard for extensive renal stones. | None recommended as first-line. |
| Lower pole stones >10 mm | Unfavorable anatomy may limit ESWL or URS success. | URS (for smaller stones). |
| Failed prior treatments | Residual fragments or inadequate clearance after ESWL or URS. | Repeat ESWL (select cases). |
| Anatomical abnormalities | Direct access to renal collecting system (e.g., horseshoe kidney). | URS (less effective in complex anatomy). |
| Cystine or hard stones | Resistant to ESWL fragmentation (e.g., calcium oxalate monohydrate). | URS with laser lithotripsy. |
| Obstructive or infected stones | Simultaneous drainage and stone clearance in cases of infection or obstruction. | Drainage (temporary) + delayed PCNL. |

**Table 1.**
*Indications for PCNL and alternative treatment.*

3. *Lower pole stones > 10 mm*: For lower pole stones of significant size, PCNL is preferred when unfavorable anatomy (e.g., steep infundibulopelvic angle) reduces the success of other modalities.

4. *Failed previous treatments*: PCNL is indicated when ESWL or URS fails to achieve satisfactory stone clearance.

5. *Anatomical abnormalities*: Patients with congenital or acquired renal anomalies (e.g., horseshoe kidney, ureteropelvic junction obstruction) benefit from PCNL as it allows direct access to the renal collecting system.

6. *Cystine or hard stones*: PCNL is particularly effective for treating cystine or calcium oxalate monohydrate stones, which are resistant to fragmentation by ESWL.

7. *Obstructive or infected stones*: In cases of obstructive pyelonephritis or infected stones with a risk of sepsis, PCNL allows for simultaneous drainage and stone removal.

The AUA and EAU guidelines emphasize that the choice of treatment should also consider patient-specific factors such as overall health, renal function, and preferences. Additionally, advanced imaging techniques, including CT urography, are critical for preoperative planning to assess stone characteristics and renal anatomy, further refining the indication for PCNL.

## 4. Contraindications for PCNL

Although PCNL is highly effective for managing complex and large renal stones, there are specific contraindications that must be considered to ensure patient safety. According to the American Urological Association (AUA) and European Association of Urology (EAU) guidelines, these contraindications include uncorrected coagulopathy, active untreated infections, pregnancy, severe cardiorespiratory instability, non-functioning kidneys, and morbid obesity.

| Contraindication | Details |
|---|---|
| Uncorrected coagulopathy | Increased risk of bleeding; correct preoperatively. |
| Active untreated infection | High risk of sepsis; requires preoperative antibiotic therapy. |
| Pregnancy | Radiation exposure contraindicates PCNL. |
| Severe cardiorespiratory instability | Unsuitable for prone positioning or physiological stress. |
| Non-functioning kidney | No benefit from stone removal in non-functional kidneys. |
| Morbid obesity | Challenges in renal access and increased perioperative risks. |

**Table 2.**
*Contraindications for PCNL.*

Uncorrected coagulopathy significantly increases the risk of bleeding and must be managed preoperatively. Similarly, patients with active untreated infections require preoperative antibiotic therapy to reduce the risk of sepsis. Pregnant patients should avoid PCNL due to the risks associated with radiation exposure during fluoroscopy. Non-functional kidneys provide no clinical benefit from stone removal, and morbid obesity presents technical challenges for renal access and increased perioperative risks (**Table 2**).

## 5. Patient positioning in PCNL: Prone vs. supine (Valdivia-Galdakao) approach

The choice of patient positioning in percutaneous nephrolithotomy (PCNL) remains a subject of ongoing debate, with two primary approaches being predominantly utilized: the prone position and the supine Valdivia-Galdakao position. Each offers distinct advantages and limitations that influence surgical outcomes, complication rates, and procedural efficiency.

### 5.1 Prone position

The prone position has historically been the standard for PCNL, with approximately 60–70% of procedures performed this way worldwide. This position provides excellent access to the kidney, particularly the posterior calyces, and offers a larger surface area for renal puncture. Additionally, gravitational assistance helps in the clearance of stone fragments (**Figure 2**).

*Advantages of the Prone Position:*

- Improved access to the posterior calyces.

- Minimal interference from other abdominal organs.

- Reduced risk of colonic injury due to the posterior approach.

*Disadvantages:*

- Increased patient morbidity due to the need for repositioning after anesthesia induction.

- Higher risk of respiratory compromise in patients with cardiopulmonary conditions.

- More challenging for anesthesiologists to monitor and manage the airway.

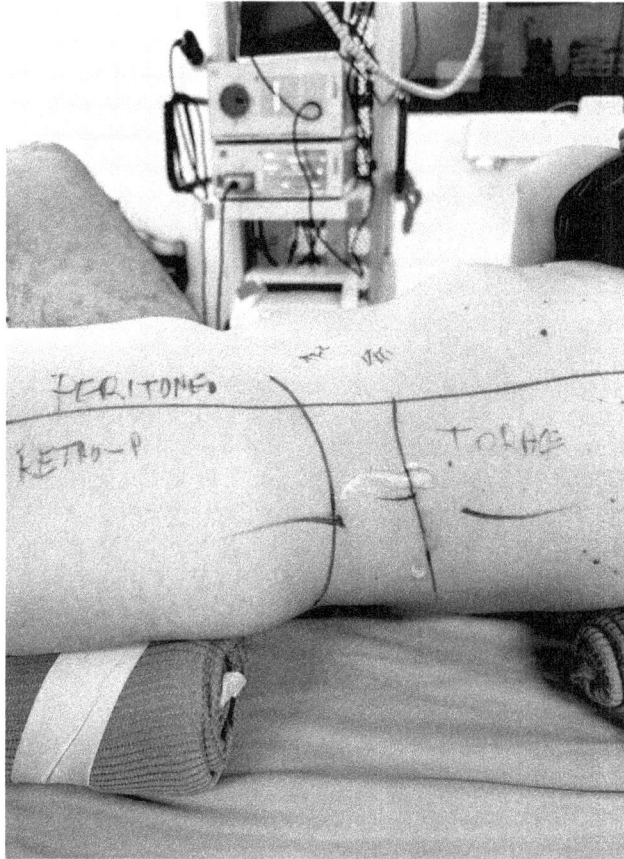

**Figure 2.**
*Anatomical references for renal puncture.*

## 5.2 Supine (Valdivia-Galdakao) position

The supine Valdivia-Galdakao position has gained popularity, now accounting for approximately 30–40% of PCNL procedures. This approach allows simultaneous retrograde access and is considered less invasive, with shorter operative times in certain contexts.

*Advantages of the Supine Position:*

- Easier airway management and hemodynamic stability.

- Facilitates combined approaches such as Endoscopic Combined Intra-Renal Surgery (ECIRS).

- Reduced operative time due to the absence of patient repositioning.

*Disadvantages:*

- Limited access to posterior calyces.

- Higher risk of bowel injury due to the anterior approach.

- Increased difficulty in puncturing the inferior calyces.

### 5.3 Comparative outcomes

Studies comparing the two positions have shown similar stone-free rates and overall complication profiles. However, the choice often depends on institutional protocols, surgeon expertise, and specific patient factors such as body habitus and comorbidities. While the prone position remains the gold standard for complex and multiple stone burdens, the supine approach is increasingly preferred for its versatility and patient safety advantages.

## 6. PCNL types based on access caliber

Different variations of PCNL exist, classified based on the caliber of the percutaneous access. The choice of technique depends on factors such as stone size and location, the patient's anatomy, and the surgeon's experience.

## 7. Instrumentation

Accurate preparation of the instrumentation and in-depth knowledge of each instrument are crucial for the success of a PCNL procedure. Proper organization and ensuring the availability of all necessary tools before the start of the surgery are critical, as the lack of a specific instrument could compromise the effectiveness of the procedure and extend the operative time, directly impacting the patient's postoperative recovery. Proper planning and efficient management of the instruments contribute to the safety and successful outcome of the surgery.

### 7.1 Radiological and access instrumentation

- *C-arm fluoroscopy* for intraoperative imaging and guidance

- *Cystoscope* for the placement of the ureteral catheter or occluding balloon

- *Pollack ureteral catheter* for renal contrast injection and dilation facilitation

- *Chiba needle* for initial renal puncture

- *Fascial dilators:*

  - *Alken metallic dilators* for controlled stepwise dilation

  - *Progressive conical dilators* for gradual tract expansion

  - *Balloon dilators* for rapid dilation with minimal tissue trauma

- *Guidewires* (hydrophilic, super stiff, nitinol core, etc.)

| Type | Access Diameter | Instrumentation Used | Advantages | Disadvantages |
|------|-----------------|----------------------|------------|---------------|
| Standard PCNL | 24–30 Fr | Rigid nephroscope, lithotripsy tools | High effectiveness for large stones | Greater tissue trauma and bleeding risk |
| Mini-PCNL | 14–20 Fr | Mini-nephroscope, laser lithotripsy | Less invasive, reduced blood loss | Slower stone fragment removal |
| Ultra-mini PCNL | 11–13 Fr | Small-caliber nephroscope, continuous aspiration | Minimally invasive, lower renal trauma | Less efficient for hard stone removal |
| Micro-PCNL | <10 Fr | Micro-nephroscope, thin fiber laser | Least invasive, suitable for small stones | Not effective for large stones |
| Super-mini PCNL | 12–14 Fr | Nephroscope with dedicated aspiration system | Good balance between efficiency and invasiveness | Requires specialized equipment |

**Table 3.**
*Different types of PCNL based on caliber.*

### 7.2 Components for nephroscope placement

- *Amplatz sheath* (or alternatives such as Clear Petra) to maintain the working channel

- *Nephroscope* in various sizes (**Table 3**)

### 7.3 Drainage and safety devices

- *Occluding balloon* to control fragment outflow

- *Dual lumen catheter* for drainage and combined irrigation or for double guide-wire placement.

- *Nephrostomy kit* with drainage catheters of appropriate caliber for the selected technique

- *Ureteral Stent Double J*

### 7.4 Energy sources for stone fragmentation

- Pneumatic lithotripsy (ballistic)

- Ultrasonic lithotripsy

- Holmium-YAG laser

## 8. PCNL procedure: From strategy to execution

The procedure begins only when the surgeon has a well-defined strategy, supported by the study of preoperative imaging. A clear plan is crucial for achieving optimal outcomes and minimizing complications.

The intervention starts with retrograde access via cystoscopy, allowing the insertion of a guidewire, typically a standard PTFE wire. In cases of a non-compliant ureter, a different type of guidewire may be required to facilitate safe and effective access. In cases of ureteral compliance, the use of a ureteral catheter with the active guidewire technique can be highly beneficial to maintain continuous flow, optimize endoscopic visualization, and reduce intrarenal pressure [6]. Through the ureteral catheter, a pyelography is performed to study the urinary tract, opacify the calyces, and distend the collecting system, making the subsequent puncture easier.

When the anatomy allows, an occluding balloon can be placed over the guidewire to maintain the dilation of the collecting system. This device also enables the opacification or irrigation of the calyceal system as needed. It is considered good practice to place a bladder catheter to avoid excessive bladder distension during the procedure.

The calyceal puncture is then performed using a 21G Chiba needle under combined ultrasound and fluoroscopic guidance. It is crucial to wait for urine efflux, confirming successful puncture of the calyx. The choice of the targeted calyx depends on the pre-established strategy to approach the stone. Most commonly, the lower or middle calyx is selected for optimal access. The puncture should be directed toward the center of the papilla to minimize bleeding, which can compromise visibility and pose a potential risk of anemia.

Once the calyx has been successfully punctured, two guidewires are positioned:

- A super stiff guidewire for operative use.

- A safety guidewire to maintain secure access in case of accidental displacement of the primary channel.

Dilation of the access tract is then performed using progressive or pneumatic dilators, allowing the placement of the working sheath. At this point, the nephroscope can be introduced along with the selected energy source and aspiration system, facilitating the removal of stone fragments and ensuring an optimal stone-free outcome.

If necessary, flexible instruments can be employed to reach residual stones located in areas that are challenging to access with a rigid nephroscope.

At the end of the procedure, a double J ureteral stent and a nephrostomy tube are positioned to ensure proper urinary drainage and monitor post-operative outcomes.

This systematic approach, from strategic planning to execution, ensures that the procedure is carried out safely and efficiently, reducing complications and improving stone-free rates.

## 9. Combined approach in PCNL: The ECIRS technique

In certain complex cases, a combined approach that integrates percutaneous nephrolithotripsy (PCNL) with ureterorenoscopy, known as Endoscopic Combined Intra-Renal Surgery (ECIRS), can be employed. This advanced technique is particularly useful for treating kidney stones that are challenging to access solely through the percutaneous route. Moreover, it facilitates a safer puncture in complex anatomical conditions and improves the stone-free rate (SFR).

## 9.1 Concept and rationale

ECIRS utilizes both antegrade and retrograde approaches, offering a dual perspective that enhances the surgeon's ability to achieve complete stone clearance in a single session. This dual-access strategy is particularly valuable in managing staghorn stones and other complex formations. By combining the strengths of PCNL and flexible ureterorenoscopy (fURS), ECIRS overcomes the limitations of each modality when used independently.

## 9.2 Advantages of ECIRS

Improved Stone-Free Rate: Using two simultaneous access points, ECIRS increases the efficiency of fragment removal, significantly reducing the likelihood of residual stones.

Safer Calyx Puncture: In complex anatomical cases, retrograde visualization with a flexible ureterorenoscope helps identify the safest calyx for puncture, minimizing the risk of vascular injury and bleeding.

Effective Management of Upper Pole Stones: Stones located in the upper calyx are notoriously difficult to reach solely through the percutaneous route. ECIRS allows these fragments to be mobilized using a flexible ureterorenoscope and relocated to the renal pelvis or lower calyx, where they can be removed via the nephroscopic tract.

Reduction of Multiple Sessions: The goal of ECIRS is to achieve complete stone removal in a single session, reducing the need for subsequent procedures and improving patient outcomes.

## 9.3 Technical considerations

Patient Positioning: ECIRS is generally performed in the modified Galdakao-Valdivia supine position, allowing simultaneous antegrade and retrograde access with greater patient stability and shorter operative times.

## 9.4 Clinical outcomes

Studies have demonstrated that ECIRS achieves a higher stone-free rate (SFR), especially in patients with staghorn stones or complex multi-calyceal stones, compared to PCNL or flexible ureterorenoscopy alone. Additionally, it is associated with a lower complication rate due to better visualization and safer puncture techniques.

## 10. Possible complications in PCNL

Percutaneous nephrolithotomy (PCNL) is a widely accepted and effective method for the treatment of renal stones. However, like all invasive procedures, it carries a potential for complications. These complications can vary in severity and are influenced by patient factors, surgeon experience, and the complexity of the case. The most common complications include hemorrhagic, infectious, respiratory, and mechanical issues, with others arising from organ injury or procedural failures.

Hemorrhagic complications remain the most frequent, with a reported incidence of transfusion requirements in 0–20% of cases. In more severe situations, embolization may be necessary to control bleeding, which occurs in 0–1.5% of cases. These bleeding complications are usually manageable, though they may occasionally necessitate surgical intervention or embolization to control significant blood loss.

Urinary leaks or urinomas, typically due to renal puncture or inadvertent injury to the renal collecting system, occur in 0–1% of cases. These collections of urine outside the renal system usually resolve with drainage, though some cases may require surgical revision. Infections, including urinary tract infections or sepsis, are encountered in approximately 0.3–1.1% of patients. These can be managed with appropriate antibiotic therapy and, in some instances, further stone clearance if infection is associated with residual fragments.

Respiratory complications related to patient positioning are also noteworthy, with an incidence ranging from 0 to 11.6% of cases. These may include atelectasis, pneumonia, or other issues related to prolonged positioning in the prone or modified lateral decubitus position during surgery. Vigilant monitoring and optimization of patient positioning can reduce these risks.

Injury to adjacent organs such as the liver, spleen, intestines, or pleura is a rare but serious complication, occurring in 0–1.7% of cases. These injuries typically require immediate surgical intervention or drainage and may impact the overall outcome of the procedure.

Occasionally, the procedure may be abandoned due to an unsuccessful renal puncture, occurring in approximately 5% of cases. In these instances, the puncture site may not provide adequate access to the renal collecting system, and the procedure is suspended to prevent further injury (**Figure 3**, **Table 4**).

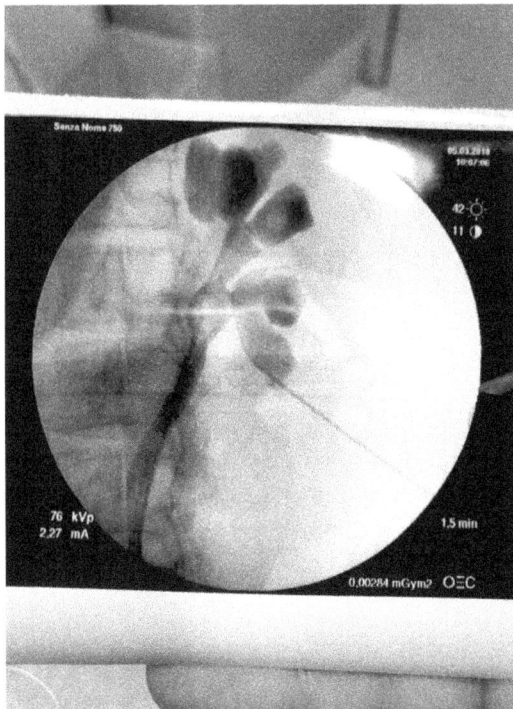

**Figure 3.**
*Example of renal puncture with radiological guidance.*

| Complication | Incidence | Management |
|---|---|---|
| Hemorrhagic Complications | 0–20% (transfusion), 0–1.5% (embolization) | Transfusion, embolization, or surgery if necessary |
| Formation of Urinoma | 0–1% | Drainage or surgical revision if necessary |
| Infectious Complications | 0.3–1.1% | Antibiotics, removal of residual fragments if necessary |
| Respiratory Complications | 0–11.6% | Monitoring and optimization of positioning |
| Injury to Perirenal Organs | 0–1.7% | Surgical intervention or drainage |
| Unsuccessful Puncture | 5% | Abandoning the procedure, possible reevaluation |

**Table 4.**
*Complications.*

## 11. Post-operative management of the patient undergoing PCNL

Accurate post-operative management is essential to ensure the success of percutaneous nephrolithotripsy (PCNL) and to promptly identify any complications.

### 11.1 First post-operative day

On the first day following the procedure, the patient is closely monitored. Routine blood tests, including complete blood count, electrolytes, and renal function parameters, are performed to assess the systemic response to the surgery and detect early signs of bleeding or renal dysfunction. If the patient is stable and no complications are apparent, the nephrostomy tube is temporarily closed to assess tolerance.

### 11.2 Second post-operative day

On the second day, if the patient reports no significant pain and the laboratory tests are within normal limits, the nephrostomy tube is removed. A plain abdominal X-ray (abdominal radiograph) is then performed to confirm the stone-free status and ensure the correct placement of the double J ureteral stent following the removal of the nephrostomy tube.

### 11.3 Discharge and follow-up

In the absence of complications, the patient is typically discharged on the fourth post-operative day. Clear instructions on post-discharge care should be provided, including pain management, fluid intake to promote urinary flow, and the eventual removal of the ureteral stent at the appropriate time. In case of persistent fever, ongoing pain, or any unusual symptoms, prompt clinical reevaluation is necessary.

## 12. Percutaneous nephrolithotomy in horseshoe kidney: Special considerations

Percutaneous nephrolithotomy (PCNL) in patients with horseshoe kidney (HSK) presents unique anatomical and surgical challenges compared to a normal kidney. The abnormal fusion of the lower poles, altered renal rotation, and aberrant vasculature require modifications in the standard approach to ensure both safety and efficacy.

Differences in Approach Compared to a Normal Kidney.

In contrast to a normal kidney, where access to the inferior calyx is often preferred for direct entry into the renal pelvis, PCNL in HSK typically favors superior calyceal access. This is due to several factors:

- Lower pole fusion and anterior displacement of the pelvis make inferior and middle calyceal punctures less favorable.

- Superior calyceal access provides a more direct and safer tract to the collecting system while reducing the risk of injuring the aberrant vasculature or adjacent structures (e.g., bowel).

- Minimized bleeding risk, as puncturing near the isthmus increases the likelihood of vascular complications.

## 13. Key surgical considerations

- *Preoperative imaging is critical*

  o Detailed preoperative CT urography and Doppler ultrasound are essential to delineate the altered anatomy, particularly vascular anomalies. This minimizes the risk of injuring aberrant arteries that frequently originate from the aorta or iliac arteries.

- *Optimal patient positioning*

  o Prone position remains the most commonly used due to better access to the superior calyces and posterior orientation of the collecting system.

  o Supine approach may be challenging because of the anteriorly displaced renal pelvis and increased risk of bowel interference.

- *Percutaneous access strategy*

  o Superior calyceal puncture is preferred to avoid complications associated with the isthmus.

  o Fluoroscopic and ultrasound-guided access is strongly recommended due to the altered renal axis.

  o Nephrostomy tract dilation should be performed cautiously, considering the increased vascularity around the isthmus.

- *Stone clearance challenges*

  o Fragments may migrate due to abnormal pelvicalyceal orientation, necessitating flexible nephroscopy or a combined approach (e.g., ECIRS).

o Drainage considerations: The altered urinary drainage pattern may require prolonged nephrostomy tube placement postoperatively.

PCNL in horseshoe kidney demands meticulous planning, superior calyceal access, and a cautious approach to vascular and visceral structures. With appropriate modifications, stone-free rates comparable to those in normal kidneys can be achieved, while minimizing the risk of complications.

## 14. Conclusion

Percutaneous nephrolithotomy (PCNL) continues to evolve as one of the cornerstone procedures for the treatment of renal stones, demonstrating exceptional outcomes in terms of success and reduced risk of complications when performed with skill and attention to detail. However, ensuring the success and safety of the procedure requires strict adherence to established protocols and guidelines, as well as thorough preparation by the surgical team. Minimally invasive techniques, coupled with the use of combinable energies such as ultrasound lithotripsy, pneumatic lithotripsy, and laser, provide versatile options to ensure the procedure's effectiveness.

Nevertheless, PCNL is not without risks, and the success of the procedure is strongly dependent on the surgeon's experience, the surgical team's preparedness, and the precision in choosing the right instruments. It is through proper planning, refining the technique, and a deep understanding of potential complications that the benefits of the procedure can be maximized.

To conclude, the "10 Commandments of PCNL" serve as a valuable guide for every surgeon embarking on this complex and delicate procedure. By following these principles, one can not only achieve a high success rate but also significantly improve patient safety and minimize the risk of complications.

*The 10 Commandments of PCNL:*

1. *Do not perform the procedure if you are not skilled enough* (the surgeon's ego has no place when patient safety is at stake)

2. *The procedure must be completed in your mind before you begin*

3. *Do not start unless you have every device you may need on the operating table*

4. *Never compromise on the instruments* (a compromise means complications or an incomplete procedure)

5. *Know the steps and master them for every eventuality*

6. *The ureter and renal pelvis are sacred; do not force them or they will make you pay*

7. *There is no indication for PCNL without a CT scan*

8. *The smaller it is, the less functional it is*

9. *Choose the right energy* (combined energy should be used)

10. *Trust in yourself*

These commandments are not merely suggestions but fundamental principles that every surgeon should follow to ensure that PCNL is performed smoothly, with the best results for the patient. Discipline, preparation, and a systematic approach are the secrets to executing this procedure successfully and safely, minimizing risks and maximizing benefits for the patient.

## Author details

Alessandro Calarco* and Pietro Viscuso
San Carlo di Nancy Hospital, Rome, Italy

*Address all correspondence to: alecalarco@gmail.com

**IntechOpen**

## References

[1] EAU Guidelines. Available from: https://uroweb.org/guidelines

[2] AUA Guidelines. Available from: https://www.auanet.org/guidelines-and-quality/guidelines

[3] Mantica G, Leonardi R, Calarco A, Senel S, Uzun E, Ceviz K, et al. predictive factors for difficult ureter in patients undergoing retrograde intrarenal surgery. The Central European Journal of Urology. 2024;**77**(3):518-519. DOI: 10.5173/ceju.2024.128. Epub 2024 Sep 30

[4] Tufano A, Frisenda M, Rossi A, Viscuso P, Mantica G, Bove P, et al. External validation of Resorlu-Unsal stone score in predicting outcomes after retrograde intrarenal surgery. Experience from a single institution. Archivio Italiano di Urologia, Andrologia. 2022;**94**(3):311-314. DOI: 10.4081/aiua.2022.3.311

[5] Sighinolfi MC, Calcagnile T, Ticonosco M, Kaleci S, Bari DIS, Assumma S, et al. External validation of a nomogram for outcome prediction in management of medium-sized (1-2 cm) kidney stones. Minerva Urology and Nephrology. 2024;**76**(4):484-490. DOI: 10.23736/S2724-6051.24.05672-6. Epub 2024 May 10

[6] Calarco A, Frisenda M, Molinaro E, Lenci N. The active guidewire technique versus standard technique as different way to approach ureteral endoscopic stone treatment. Archivio Italiano di Urologia, Andrologia. 2021;**93**(4):431-435. DOI: 10.4081/aiua.2021.4.431

# Iterative Process in Nephrolithiasis Management: A Focus on Translational Approach

*John Emenike Anieche, Chukwuka Azubuike*
*and Ngozi Eucheria Makata*

## Abstract

Nephrolithiasis is both clinical and public health concerned disease referred to as presence of concretions in the urinary system. Location, composition, and sizes of stones vary. Diagnosis, treatment, and prevention of nephrolithiasis have diverse approaches with the primary aim of reduction of symptoms and its effect on the patient. The approach taken for the treatment depends on the knowledge of the MD and preferences. To facilitate a faster, more responsive, timely, and less expensive treatment of this disease, a translational approach remains an option to go by. It is a means by which biomedical and public health research helps improve the health of patients by translating research findings into diagnostic tools, procedures, and policies about the disease. This bridges the gap between preclinical research and clinical applications that could cure the diseases, which involve the use of biomarkers and artificial intelligence to hasten the diagnosis and application of well-defined measures for the treatment.

**Keywords:** nephrolithiasis, advances, treatment, translational, approaches

## 1. Introduction

Nephrolithiasis describes a syndrome characterized by the development of solid crystalline masses within the urinary space of the kidney [1]. The initial precipitation forms a nucleus or matrix that promotes further precipitation and calculus enlargement [2].

Sometimes the stones will be of mixed composition. For instance, calcium and oxalate, phosphate and oxalate may form stone [3]. Sizes as well as shapes of the stones vary. Urinary stones can form anywhere in the urinary tract, and they bear their names according to their location or element (s) that formed them. For instance, stone in the kidney is referred to as kidney stone; stone in the ureter is called ureteral stone; and stone in the bladder is referred to as bladder stone. Stones may be developed in one or both kidneys [4].

If stone is formed by calcium, it can be called "calcium stone"; if it is formed by uric acid, it can be called "uric acid stone" [5]. There is a specialized type of stone known as staghorn calculus, which is composed of struvite (calcium phosphate) often located at the renal pelvis but extends to the calyces.

IntechOpen

The pain that comes with nephrolithiasis is often accompanied by nausea, vomiting, and malaise; fever and chills may be present. Treatment of nephrolithiasis varies and depends on the causative factor, but generally increased fluid intake is often advocated [6].

## 1.1 Endoscopic removal or surgery are other options

The above treatment measures notwithstanding, preventive measures that involve a combination of lifestyle maintenance of healthy weight, dietary modification, and exercise will yield positive outcomes [7, 8]. In order to ensure better treatment outcomes, the need for translational approach cannot be overemphasized as integration of knowledge from various disciplines arising from research outcomes will definitely yield the most expected outcome among the patients.

## 2. Epidemiology of nephrolithiasis

Nephrolithiasis globally occurs in 7–13% of the North American population, 5–9% of Europeans, and 1–5% of Asians. The disease depends on aspects like feeding habits, climatic conditions, and heredity; increased incidence is blamed on changes in lifestyle and global warming [9].

The prevalence of nephrolithiasis is 10.6% for males and 7.1% for females; however, recent studies show that the rate is increasing among women, with estimates that the ratio of affected males to females is 1:3:1 [10].

Age is one of the main risk factors, with a high incidence peak at 30–60 years of age.

Recurrent incidences of the condition are common, and research shows that approximately half of patients who develop a kidney stone will develop another within a period of 5 to 10 years. Conditions like high volumes of dietary sodium or salts, low volumes of water intake, or diets that contain a lot of animal protein contribute a lot to the formation of the stones. Further, climatic factors are involved; warm climate increases dehydration and concentrated urine, hence high prevalence rates in warmer climates [11].

Other risk factors include:

- Chronic urinary tract infections

- Concentration of the constituents of urine

- Hyperparathyroidism (due to increased calcium metabolism)

- Excessive ingestion of Vitamin D

- Excessive ingestion of milk or an alkali such as magnesium trisilicate.

- Prolonged immobilization (this gives room for matrix formation and concentration of urine)

- Diet high in animal protein

- Antibiotics, protease inhibitors, and certain diuretics cause the risk of kidney stones

- An analogous effect may occur in the case of obesity or weight loss associated with laxative misuse, rapid depletion of muscle tissue, or inadequate hydration [12].


## 3. Types of kidney stones

Nephrolithiasis or more commonly known as kidney stones are mineral concretions found inside the kidneys [13]. These stones differ in composition, and therefore, various types that include the cause and treatment of each type may also be different. Below are the primary types of kidney stones:

1. Calcium stone: Calcium stones are the most frequent, approximately 80% of kidney stones are composed of calcium oxalate, with smaller percentages consisting of calcium phosphate or a mixture of both. It also identifies risk factors such as hypercalciuria, dietary influences, and reduced water intake leading to dehydration. The cause of its development specifically includes hypercalciuria, renal as well as dietary factors, and reduced water intake leading to dehydration [14].

2. Struvite stones: Struvite stones are particularly common in patients suffering from an infection with bacteria that split urea in the urinary tract, thus increasing the pH of the urine. These stones are formed by magnesium ammonium phosphate and have a tendency to grow large, and they may produce staghorn calculi [15].

3. Uric acid stone: Uric acid nephrolithiasis, a form of kidney stone disease, results from the accumulation of uric acid crystals in the kidneys. These crystals can aggregate into stones, leading to painful and potentially recurrent urinary tract obstructions. This condition often correlates with elevated uric acid levels in the bloodstream, known as hyperuricemia. Almost two-thirds of all uric acid kidney stones can be dissolved by increasing urinary pH and volume and decreasing hyperuricosuria [16].

4. Cystine stones: Cystine stones are less common, and cystine is formed due to a hereditary condition called cystinuria. Cystinuria is an inherited disorder of the dibasic amino acid transport system in the proximal tubule and the small intestine. Two responsible genes have been identified, the SLC3A1 on chromosome 2 and the SLC7A9 on chromosome 19. The inability of renal tubules to reabsorb cystine and the relative insolubility of cystine at physiological urine pH lead to stone formation [17].

5. Mixed stones: Many renal calculi are formed from a mixture of constituents, for instance, calcium oxalate and uric acid. Compositional variations might occur because of common endocrine and metabolic gamble and stone characteristics [15].

## 4. Incidence

- Occurs more in older adults and men.

- More common in people suffering from certain diseases such as short bowel syndrome (short gut), malabsorption syndrome disorder caused by a lack of functional small intestine, which manifests with diarrhea, dehydration, and malnutrition.

- People who do not take enough water.

## 5. Diagnostic investigations of nephrolithiasis

Organized imaging is crucial in the diagnosis and assessment of nephrolithiasis for appropriate management. Different imaging techniques are used to determine the location, size, and nature of stone.

Below are the commonly used imaging techniques:

### 5.1 Non-contrast computed tomography or also called non-contrast computed tomography (NCCT)

This is the most accurate test when diagnosing nephrolithiasis because of its high sensitivity and specificity. They are able to identify stones as small as 1–2 mm and offer information on stone size, position, and quantity. This modality is very valuable in revealing the radiolucent stone, like uric acid stone, which may not be seen on ordinary X-ray film. Nevertheless, it has shortcomings like radiation hazards and increased expense [18].

### 5.2 Ultrasound (US)

Sonography is a common modality for imaging that is employed in primary assessments and subsequent checkups. It is, however, more preferred in pediatric and pregnant patients since it does not cause ionizing radiation. This notwithstanding, as an imaging modality, ultrasound is more specific for identifying laparoscopic access larger stones and hydronephrosis but is less specific for the identification of small or ureteral stones [19].

### 5.3 Plain radiography (KUB)

KUB radiography is coated, inexpensive, and easily accessible most of the time. It is most helpful for following the position of radiopaque stones during follow-up. However, its sensitivity is lower compared to NCCT; it will not be able to identify radiolucent stones or stones that are superimposed by bony structures [20].

### 5.4 Magnetic resonance imaging (MRI)

As an imaging study, MRI is not frequently employed in nephrolithiasis, but may be helpful in certain special circumstances, such as pregnancy or conditions that exclude the use of radiation. MRI is invaluable in visualizing soft tissue, but it is not so helpful in identifying calcified stones [21].

## 5.5 Intravenous urography (IVU)

In the past, intravenous urography (IVU) was the definitive diagnostic modality for evaluating stones, but with the introduction of non-contrast CT (NCCT). It employs contrast agents to help display the urinary tract, and therefore, the examinations are valuable in functional evaluations. However, its sensitivity and specificity are comparatively lower than the NCCT, and the risk of contrast-related complications is involved [22].

## 5.6 Dual-energy CT (DECT)

DECT is relatively new and can distinguish between different types of stone material—uric acid and calcium. This capability must hold when designing treatment approaches, as the patient's sex should also come into play here. However, its availability is relatively low, and the procedure is associated with increased radiation levels compared to regular CT [23].

## 5.7 Laboratory investigations of nephrolithiasis

Serologic and urine laboratory tests have great importance in diagnosis, evaluation, and prevention of nephrolithiasis. These investigations are to discover the causes of formation of stones, to analyze the composition of the stones, and to look at metabolic changes.

## 5.8 Urinalysis

Renal stone assessment is anchored by urinalysis. A simple dipstick test result or microscopic examination of urine sample can reveal behaviors such as hematuria, pyuria, or crystalluria—all of which are characteristic of renal calculi. The last value is crucial because the values below 5.5 indicate the presence of uric acid stone, while the values exceeding 7.5 point to struvite infection stone.

## 5.9 Stone analysis

The determination of the chemical nature of a passed or a removed stone is invaluable in kind and preventive approach toward the type of stone. These are most generally calcium oxalate, calcium phosphate, uric acid, struvite, and cystine stones [24].

## 5.10 Serum studies

Serum calcium: Hypercalcemia may be due to primary hyperparathyroidism, a cause of calcium-containing stones.

- Serum uric acid: High amounts are related to formation of the uric acid stone or gout.

- Renal function tests: These evaluate the effects of stones on renal function [25].

## 5.11 24-hour urine collection

A comprehensive 24-hour urine analysis evaluates risk factors for stone formation, including:

- Urinary volume: How much urine does a patient make in 24 hours should be an area of interest as this helps to estimate the functional state of the kidneys. Urine calcium, oxalate, citrate, uric acid, and sodium levels are expressed as mass per area, along with supersaturation indices for stone-forming salts.

This test is particularly applicable for recurrent stone formers or history of having nephrolithiasis in the family [26].

### 5.12 Microbiological studies

In patients who are suspected to have infection-related stones, urine culture is mandatory to control the organisms. Infection stones are considered to be created by the urease-producing bacteria including *Proteus mirabilis* [25].

### 5.13 Genetic testing

If the stone formation is recurrent or if the patient with nephrolithiasis develops stones at a young age, some rare inherited metabolic disorders like cystinuria or primary hyperoxaluria may be diagnosed by genetic screening [27].

## 6. Pathological effects of nephrolithiasis

Formation of stone (calculus) in any part of the urinary system will obstruct the normal flow of urine. Smaller or tiny stones may be symptomless [28].

If the stone is not flushed out, it will cause referred pain, which is felt in the flank and groin. Pressure from stone on the tiny blood vessels in the membrane covering the structure may rupture, leading to bleeding (hematuria) [29].

Several pathological effects may occur on the kidneys and urinary tract, which include:

- Hydronephrosis: Prolonged obstruction can cause the kidney to swell, leading to hydronephrosis, which can impair kidney function.

- Pyelonephritis: Bacterial infections can occur in the presence of kidney stones, leading to pyelonephritis, a type of kidney infection.

- Interstitial nephritis: Chronic inflammation and scarring can occur in the kidney tissue, leading to interstitial nephritis.

- Renal parenchymal damage: Repeated episodes of kidney stones can cause damage to the renal parenchyma, leading to scarring and impaired kidney function.

- Chronic kidney disease: Untreated or recurrent kidney stones can increase the risk of developing chronic kidney disease.

- Hypercalciuria: Excessive calcium in the urine can lead to kidney stones and metabolic bone disease.

- Hypokalemia: Low potassium levels can occur due to excessive potassium loss in the urine.

- Metabolic acidosis: Kidney stones can cause metabolic acidosis, a condition that indicates an excess amount of acid in the blood due to dysfunctional kidneys.

- Fever and chills: These may suggest a co-existent urinary tract infection (UTI) or pyelonephritis, which can be contributory to nephrolithiasis

- Kidney failure: Kidney stones are a significant and independent risk factor for kidney disease, with the prevalence of 9.6% and a 5-year recurrent rate of 37.7% observed in Taiwan [30].

- Cardiovascular disease: Studies have shown that nephrolithiasis is associated with the risk of cardiovascular disease. This is because some shared risk factors, such as hypertension, obesity, oxidative stress, and others, may occur as off-shoot of kidney stone. Early diagnosis and treatment of nephrolithiasis are essential to prevent these pathological effects and complications.

## 7. Conventional treatment of nephrolithiasis

Tiny and disintegrated stones may be passed out through the urine, and therefore, inspection of every urine sample to detect stone is important. Ensure that all urine passes through gauze because some stones such as uric acid stones may break into pieces. Once the stone is flushed, no other treatment is required, but the patient may still continue with high fluid intake for a few days [2].

Dietary restriction is also used in some cases of management, but this depends on the substance(s) that formed the stone. If the core content of the stone is calcium, low calcium and Vit. D in diet should be served to the client. If it was formed by calcium phosphate, the urine is made acidic by drinking 3–4 glasses of cranberry juice daily, a wild red edible berry, which helps to dissolve the stones, and they are passed out through the urine [2]. Uric acid stone is treated by making the urine alkaline through the use of a sodium citrate or bicarbonate mixture to dissolve the stone.

Uric acid stone is treated by making the urine alkaline through the use of a sodium citrate or bicarbonate mixture to dissolve the stone [31]. Note that most stones are of mixed composition, and sometimes dietary restrictions may not solve the problem. Pain can be managed using analgesics such as NSAID like Ibuprofen, which reduces pain by preventing prostaglandin synthesis. If the pain is severe, opioid analgesics may be the drug of choice. Allopurinol may be prescribed to lower the serum uric acid level, especially in uric acid stone. Large stones that cause obstruction can be removed through a surgical procedure [32].

## 8. Advances in the treatment of nephrolithiasis

Advances in the treatment of nephrolithiasis have contributed a lot to the management of the disease. The application of minute or minimal invasive treatment has become highly acceptable as the need for open surgery has been reduced [33]. The type of surgery depends on the location of the stone, viz.: [34].

- Stone in the kidney—Nephrolithotomy or nephrectomy = removal of renal calculus by incising the kidney

- Stone in the renal pelvis—Pyelolithotomy = surgical removal of stone from renal pelvis

- Stone in the ureter—Ureterolithotomy = removal of calculus in the ureter.

## 9. Translational approach in nephrolithiasis treatment

Translational medicine has been defined as a discipline within biomedical and public health research that helps improve the health of individuals and the community by translating findings into diagnostic tools, medicines, procedures, policies, and education [35]. It helps to facilitate a faster, easier, more fluid, more responsive, more timely, and less expensive transition between preclinical medical research and clinical applications that could cure diseases in humans.

The purpose of the translational approach is to facilitate a faster, easier, more responsive, timely, and less expensive transition between preclinical medical research and clinical applications that could cure diseases in humans. It involves the application of basic scientific research to clinical practice with the goal of improving patient outcomes. It is a process of turning observations in the laboratory, clinic, and the community into actions that will improve the health of individuals. The conventional approach of treating nephrolithiasis ignores patient-specific requirements because they continue using a one-size-fits-all methodology [36].

The therapy known as shockwave lithotripsy proves beneficial for particular patients, although it results in secondary complications as well as stone reoccurrence [37]. Medical drugs including potassium citrate act to stop stone development yet cause undesirable side effects and react with different medications [38]. Individualized treatment strategies form another advantage of utilizing a translational approach in nephrolithiasis management. Translational research uses knowledge of distinct genetic profiles and patient-specific environmental aspects together with disease presentation to individualize treatments [36]. By performing genetic tests, medical professionals can discover which patients possess certain gene mutations creating elevated nephrolithiasis susceptibility [39]. This information can be used to develop targeted prevention and treatment strategies, which may improve patient outcomes and reduce the risk of complications.

Using translational methods in nephrolithiasis treatment enables the development of both upgraded diagnostic equipment and testing biomarkers for the condition. Advanced technologies including genomics and proteomics allow translational research to discover new biomarkers for interpreting nephrolithiasis assessment [40].

These biomarkers enable medical detection of the disease during its early phases of development, where medical interventions prove more effective, along with tracking both disease evolution and treatment effects.

The conditions that affect treatment success emphasize the requirement for a tailored method in treating nephrolithiasis, whereas translational approaches to nephrolithiasis treatment integrate basic scientific research, clinical expertise, and patient-centered care to develop innovative, effective, and personalized treatment strategies. By applying advanced technologies, such as genomics, proteomics, and metabolomics, translational research can identify novel biomarkers, therapeutic targets, and disease mechanisms [40]. For example, genetic testing can identify patients with specific mutations that increase their risk of developing nephrolithiasis [39]. This information can be used to develop targeted prevention and treatment strategies, which may improve patient outcomes and reduce the risk of complications.

## 10. Roles of biomarkers in diagnosis and prognosis

Biomarkers are measurable indicators of biological processes or pharmacological responses to therapeutic interventions [41]. The use of biomarkers arises as indispensable tools in the diagnosis and prognosis of disorders including nephrolithiasis. Thus, biomarkers are very important tools in diagnosing, predicting the course of, and treating nephrolithiasis (kidney stones). They give information about the nature of the disease process, inform management of the disease, and help in prognosis.

### 10.1 Biomarkers for diagnosis

*10.1.1 Urinary biomarkers*

Urine biomarkers are essential in measuring substances in urine, such as calcium and uric acid, and therefore, they can be used in the analysis and identification of metabolic abnormalities associated with stone formation:

- Calcium: Hypercalciuria itself has an important connection with the formation of calcium-containing stones.

- Oxalate: High urinary oxalate is associated with the formation of calcium oxalate crystals and hence stone formation.

- Citrate: Hypocitraturia diminishes the person's capacity to prevent crystal accumulation [42].

- Uric acid: Hyperuricosuria leads to the formation of uric acid stones. In contrast, a urine pH above 7 favors the formation of calcium phosphate stones [43].

*10.1.2 Serum biomarkers*

This is used in measuring substances in the blood, such as creatinine and urea. This helps in the assessment of kidney function and easy diagnosis of nephrolithiasis. Blood tests help identify systemic conditions contributing to stone formation:

- Parathyroid hormone (PTH): High PTH indicates hyperparathyroidism, which is a cause of hypercalciuria.

- Creatinine: Assesses renal function that may determine the formation of stone.

- Vitamin D: High concentration was known to raise levels of calcium and phosphorus reabsorption and excretion [44].

*10.1.3 Genetic biomarkers*

Nephrolithiasis is also passed through an autosomal recessive inherited basis due to mutations in genes such as SLC34A1 or CLCN5 to help pinpoint susceptible populations [45].

*10.1.4 Imagine biomarkers*

This is the use of imaging techniques such as ultrasound and CT scan to diagnose and monitor nephrolithiasis.

## 10.2 Biomarkers for prognosis

*10.2.1 Recurrence prediction*

Urinary supersaturation: Evaluates solute concentrations as a measure of crystal formation probability [43].

- Tamm-Horsfall protein (THP): THP prevents crystal aggregation, and its level may serve as an indicator of stone recurrence [46].

*10.2.2 Inflammatory markers*

C-reactive protein (CRP): High baseline concentrations of CRP show inflammation and have worse outcomes in patients with infection-related stones [47].

## 10.3 Emerging biomarkers

*10.3.1 Proteomics and metabolomics*

Biomarkers have been recently established using sophisticated technologies, such as the discovery of urinary peptides and metabolites, which enhance the understanding of stone formation's pathogenesis [48].

## 11. Usefulness of biomarkers in nephrolithiasis

- Early diagnosis: the likelihood of stone can be determined easily and early with biomarkers, thereby giving room for early treatment and prevention of possible complications.

- Prediction of presence of stone in the urinary system: the likelihood of stone formation in an individual is determined through biomarkers, making it possible to initiate preventive measures as soon as possible.

- Monitoring responses to treatment: effectiveness of treatment can be monitored through biomarkers, and room for adjustment is made where necessary.

- Used in narrowing down treatment in individuals: Treatment is tailored according to individual need and based on unique factors, thereby reducing generality of treatment.

## 12. Use of artificial intelligence in diagnosis and treatment of nephrolithiasis

Artificial intelligence algorithms can be used to analyze large datasets such as electronic health records, imaging studies, and laboratory results for the possible prediction of chances of kidney stone formation [49].

### 12.1 Diagnosis

AI enhances the identification and characterization of kidney stones through advanced imaging and data analysis:

### 12.2 Imaging analysis

Deep learning approaches are used to analyze CT scans, ultrasounds, and X-rays with great accuracy. There are numerous types of stones; based on imaging features, AI can predict efficiently calcium oxalate, uric acid, and other types of stones. Computer-aided detection of stones minimizes the likelihood of misdiagnosis and also lowers the burden of reporting on radiologists [50].

### 12.3 Prediction models

They extend that using the patient data concerning genetics, metabolic patterns, and other factors, AI can estimate the chances of formation of a stone. The cognitive methods involve feature detection for potential risks and proposing ways to avoid them [51].

### 12.4 Treatment planning

AI assists in developing personalized treatment strategies:

*12.4.1 Stone composition prediction*

In clinical applications, AI models can identify the risks of stone composition from the history and imaging data to make medical or surgical treatment decisions [52].

### 12.5 Treatment optimization

Decision-making in surgery is assisted by AI, and this leads to recommendations on the treatment intervention to be used; SWL, URS, or PCNL are dependent on size, location, and other factors. Prognostic models estimate the effects that both treatments and therapy-related adverse events will have [53].

### 12.6 Minimally invasive techniques

AI robotic systems enhance accuracy in operations, minimize adverse effects to the patient, and decrease the length of hospital stays [54].

### 12.7 Recurrence prediction

AI models predict the likelihood of stone recurrence so as to manage the matter effectively. Wearable devices in combination with AI monitor hydration status and diet and other risky factors in real time [51].

### 12.8 Telemedicine

AI-based telemedicine helps in continuous supervision of further changes in behavior and follow-up programmes [54].

### 12.9 Personalized medicine

AI helps to align treatment to an individual patient's unique medical history and lifestyle-based factors. This is achieved through the analysis of large files, including unstructured clinical notes, medical imaging reports, and others, to extract relevant information. With this, errors in medical documentation are reduced, and personalized patient care is achieved. Personalized intervention such as customized dietary changes based on the gut microbiota may improve stone prevention and recurrence [55].

### 12.10 Research and drug development

AI accelerates research into nephrolithiasis. AI-powered genomic analysis can be of help in the identification of variants that are associated with nephrolithiasis.

### 12.11 Drug discovery

AI recognizes therapeutic biomarkers and the effectiveness of novel drugs for the prevention or dissolution of the stone [50].

### 12.12 Dietary modifications

Evidence supports dietary adjustments as a cornerstone of nephrolithiasis prevention [56]. Increasing fluid intake to achieve a daily urine output of at least 2.5 liters remains a primary recommendation [57]. Water is the preferred choice, but citrus beverages like lemonade may also be beneficial due to their citrate content, which inhibits stone formation [38]. Increased water intake will help to dilute the concentration of stone-forming substances.

The risk of calcium oxalate stone formation is reduced by reduction of calcium intake. Low-calcium diets are no longer universally recommended, as adequate calcium intake can bind oxalate in the gut and reduce oxalate absorption [58]. Specific dietary strategies, including reducing sodium intake, can help in the reduction of calcium oxalate stone formation [59].

Limiting animal protein intake can help in the reduction of uric acid stone formation. Also, increasing consumption of fruits and vegetables rich in citrate helps inhibit stone formation [60]. It can be of help to increase citrate intake as citrate helps to reduce formation of kidney stone.

In light of the above, translational approach requires that patients' dietary plan be personalized and geared toward increasing substances that reduce the risk of stone formation and reducing those substances that potentiate stone formation.

### 12.13 Pharmacological interventions

Pharmacological approaches have evolved to include tailored treatments based on stone composition and patient metabolic evaluation. For calcium oxalate stones, thiazide diuretics reduce urinary calcium excretion, while potassium citrate increases urinary citrate levels, effectively reducing recurrence risk [61]. Allopurinol remains a key intervention for patients with hyperuricosuria, while newer agents targeting urate metabolism are under investigation [62].

### 12.14 Technological innovations in risk assessment

Advances in imaging and laboratory technologies have improved the precision of nephrolithiasis risk assessment. Dual-energy CT scans now enable differentiation between stone types, facilitating targeted preventive measures [63]. Furthermore, metabolomic and genomic profiling hold promise for identifying individuals at high risk, enabling personalized prevention strategies [64].

### 12.15 Gut microbiome modulation

Emerging research highlights the role of the gut microbiome in oxalate metabolism. Probiotics such as *Oxalobacter formigenes* show potential in reducing urinary oxalate excretion and stone recurrence [65]. Ongoing clinical trials aim to validate these findings and explore other microbiome-targeted therapies.

### 12.16 Behavioral and digital interventions

Behavioral strategies supported by digital tools, such as smartphone applications, have gained traction in recent years. These tools help track hydration, dietary intake, and medication adherence, empowering patients to actively participate in prevention efforts [66].

## 13. Application of translational approach to achieve better outcome in nephrolithiasis treatment

The success of translational approach in the treatment of nephrolithiasis is dependent on the applicability of the different measures implicit in the approach. To achieve this, the under-listed are indispensable.

- Interdisciplinary collaboration: Basic scientists, clinicians, and organizations should collaborate in translational research and utilization of outcomes for the good of the patients.

- Working with patient advocacy group to increase public awareness on kidney stone disease.

- The need to partner with organizations to develop the most efficient, sustainable treatment modality for nephrolithiasis will not be overemphasized.

- Personalized medical practice using genetic and metabolic profiles to streamline treatment to individual patients should be an option to follow.

- The need to analyze large datasets to assist in predicting the chances of kidney stone formation on patients will be of great value in the treatment of nephrolithiasis.

- There is a need to develop an AI-powered decision support system to give timely diagnosis and treatment.

- Dietary modifications that can assist in the prevention of kidney stones and adequate hydration should be seen as a public necessity and the campaign taken to the public.

## 14. Challenges in the application of translational approach in the treatment of nephrolithiasis

The benefits of translational approach in nephrolithiasis are numerous, but this does not mean that there are no challenges in the application of the approach. The challenges cut across scientific, clinical, regulatory, technological, and collaborative in nature.

The following challenges have been identified:

- Lack of clear guidelines for management of urinary stones in some patients.

- There is no straightforward answer to the right technique in retrograde intra-renal surgery (RIRS) rather the right planning based on the anatomy of the kidney in terms of vascularity and drainage, stone size, density, and available expertise [67].

- Complexity of nephrolithiasis: This is a complex disease with multiple genetic, lifestyle, and environmental involvement. This complex nature affects the translational approach in the treatment.

- It has been difficult to develop an effective treatment for the disease due to the heterogeneous nature of the patients affected by the disease.

- The disease has high chances of recurrence, which may be linked to difficulty in predicting the nature of patients that will develop the stones.

- Poor application of personalized approach in the treatment is an issue of concern.

- Approving new treatment modality may be very complex task due to regulatory bottlenecks cum intellectual property issues, thereby affecting the translational approach.

- Funding for research and development of new treatment modality may not be easily achieved.

- Advances in technology and their applications, such as AI and machine learning, may not be readily available worldwide, which will have a negative effect in the translational approach.

## 15. Conclusion

Treatment and prevention of nephrolithiasis have shifted from conventional treatment toward a multidisciplinary and personalized approach, leveraging advancements in nutrition science, pharmacology, and technology. Ongoing research into the microbiome and digital health tools promises further innovations, improving outcomes for individuals at risk of kidney stone disease. The application and success of translational approach in the treatment of nephrolithiasis cannot be successfully done without looking inward on the means of surmounting the challenges which cut across scientific, clinical, regulatory, technological, and collaborative spheres. The public, the patients, and the policymakers in the healthcare system have roles to play to achieve this.

## Acknowledgements

The authors acknowledge the use of Humanizer (AI tool) for language polishing of the manuscript.

## Author details

John Emenike Anieche*, Chukwuka Azubuike and Ngozi Eucheria Makata
Department of Nursing Science, Nnamdi Azikiwe University, Awka, Nigeria

*Address all correspondence to: je.anieche@unizik.edu.ng

IntechOpen

# References

[1] Shastri S, Patel J, Sambandam KK, Lederer ED. Kidney stone pathophysiology, evaluation and management: Core curriculum 2023. American Journal of Kidney Diseases. 2023;**82**(5):617-634. DOI: 10.1053/j.ajkd.2023.03.017

[2] Hinkle JL, Cheever KH. Brunner and Suddarth's Textbook of Medical-Surgical Nursing. 14th ed. Philadelphia, PA: Wolter Klower; 2022

[3] Davidson S. In: Boom NA, College NR, Walker BR, editors. Davidson's Principles and Practice of Medicine. 24th ed. Edinburgh: Churchill Livingstone Elsevier; 2023

[4] Norris TL. Porth's Pathophysiology. Concepts of Altered Health State. 10th ed. Philadelphia, PA: Wolters Kluwer; 2019

[5] Binstock MA, Ringdahl E. Diagnosis and initial management of kidney stones. American Family Physician. 2019;**99**(8):490-496. Available from: https://www.aafp.org/pubs/afp/issues/2019/0415/p490.html

[6] Dave CN. Nephrolithiasis Treatment and Management. 2023. Available from: https://emedicine.medscape.com/article/437096-treatment

[7] Smith AD, Preminger GM. Smith's Urology. New York: McGraw-Hill Education; 2017

[8] Bhojani N, Lingeman JE. Shockwave lithotripsy–new concepts and optimizing treatment parameters. The Urologic Clinics of North America. 2013;**40**(1):59-66. DOI: 10.1016/j.ucl.2012.09.001

[9] Sorokin I, Mamoulakis C, Miyazawa K, Rodgers A, Talati J, Lotan Y. Epidemiology of stone disease across the world. World Journal of Urology. 2017;**35**(9):1301-1320. DOI: 10.1007/s00345-017-2008-6

[10] Roudakova K, Monga M. The evolving epidemiology of stone disease. Indian Journal of Urology. 2014;**30**(1):44-48. DOI: 10.4103/0970-1591.124206

[11] Romero V, Akpinar H, Assimos DG. Kidney stones: A global picture of prevalence, incidence, and associated risk factors kidney stones: A global perspective. Reviews Urology. 2010;**12**:e86-e96. Available from: https://www.ncbi.nlm.nih.gov/pmc/articles/PMC2931286

[12] Ma Y, Cheng C, Jian Z, Wen J, Xiang L, Li H, et al. Risk factors for nephrolithiasis formation: An umbrella review. International Journal of Surgery. 2024;**110**:42. Available from: https://journals.lww.com/international-journal-of-surgery/fulltext/2024/09000/risk_factors_for_nephrolithiasis_formation__an.42.aspx

[13] Mayo Clinic Staff. Kidney Stones — Symptoms and Causes [Internet]. Rochester (MN): Mayo Clinic; 2024. Available from: https://www.mayoclinic.org/diseases-conditions/kidney-stones/symptoms-causes/syc-20355755 [Accessed: April 10, 2025]

[14] Alelign T, Petros B. Kidney stone disease: An update on current concepts. Advances in Urology. 2018;**2018**:3068365. DOI: 10.1155/2018/3068365

[15] Pearle MS, Calhoun EA, Curhan GC. Urolithiasis. In: Wein JF, Kavoussi LR, Partin AW, Peters CA, editors. Campbell Walsh Urology. 12th ed. Philadelphia: Elsevier; 2019. pp. 1265-1289

[16] Manish KC, Leslie SW. Uric Acid Nephrolithiasis [Internet]. Treasure Island (FL): Stat Pearls Publishing; 2023. Available from: https://www.ncbi.nlm.nih.gov/books/NBK560726 [Accessed: April 13, 2025]

[17] Saravakos P, Kokkinou V, Giannatos E. Cystinuria: Current diagnosis and management. Urology. 2014;**83**:693-699. DOI: 10.1016/j.urology.2013.10.013

[18] Kenney PJ, MD. Computed tomography evaluation of urinary lithiasis. Radiologic Clinics of North America. 2003;**41**(5):965-980. DOI: 10.1016/S0033-8389(03)00067-8

[19] Mahmud S, Abbas TO, Chowdhury MEH, Mushtak A, Kabir S, Muthiyal S, et al. Automated grading of prenatal hydronephrosis severity from segmented ultrasound images using deep learning. Expert Systems with Applications. 2024;**252**(Pt B):124594. DOI: 10.1016/j.eswa.2024.124594

[20] Al-Shawi MM, Aljama NA, Aljedani R, Alsaleh MH, Atyia N, Alsedrah A, et al. The role of radiological imaging in the diagnosis and treatment of urolithiasis: A narrative review. Cureus. 2022;**14**(12):e33041. DOI: 10.7759/cureus.33041

[21] Chow GK, Patterson DE, Blute ML, Segura JW. Ureteroscopy: Effect of technology and technique on clinical practice. The Journal of Urology. 2003;**170**(1):99-102. DOI: 10.1097/01.ju.0000070883.44091.24

[22] Shine S. Urinary calculus: IVU vs. CT renal stone? A critically appraised topic. Abdominal Imaging. 2008;**33**(1):41-43. DOI: 10.1007/s00261-007-9307-0

[23] Stępień M, Chrzan R, Gawlas W. In vitro analysis of urinary stone composition in dual-energy computed tomography. Polish Journal of Radiology. 2018;**83**:e421-e425. DOI: 10.5114/pjr.2018.79588

[24] Rajendran S, Thiruppathi K, Sundaram R, Krishnan S. Bio-chemical analysis and FTIR-spectral studies of artificially removed urinary stones. Journal of Minerals and Materials Characterization and Engineering. 2009;**8**(2):115-125. Available from: https://www.scirp.org/pdf/JMMCE20090200007_26019485.pdf

[25] Wollin DA, Kaplan AG, Preminger GM, Ferraro PM, Nouvenne A, Tasca A, et al. Defining metabolic activity of nephrolithiasis – Appropriate evaluation and follow-up of stone formers. Asian Journal of Urology. 2018;**5**(4):235-242. DOI: 10.1016/j.ajur.2018.06.007

[26] Ferraro PM, Taylor EN, Curhan GC. 24-hour urinary chemistries and kidney stone risk. American Journal of Kidney Diseases. 2024;**84**(2):164-169. DOI: 10.1053/j.ajkd.2024.03.005

[27] Monico CG, Milliner DS. Genetic determinants of urolithiasis. Nature Reviews. Nephrology. 2012;**8**(3):151-162. DOI: 10.1038/nrneph.2011.211

[28] Merck Manuals. Stones in the Urinary Tract. Available from: https://www.merckmanuals.com/home/kidney-and-urinary-tract-disorders/stones-in-the-urinary-tract/stones-in-the-urinary-tract

[29] Wikipedia Contributors. Kidney Stone Disease. Wikipedia. Available from: https://en.wikipedia.org/wiki/Kidney_stone_disease [Accessed: April 14, 2025]

[30] Wu S, Shen J, Mau K, Lee Y, Chen H, Chen Y, et al. An emerging model to

screen potential medicinal plants for nephrolithiasis, an independent risk factor for chronic kidney disease. Evidence-Based Complementary and Alternative Medicine. 2014;**2014**:972958. DOI: 10.1155/2014/972958

[31] Türk C, Petřík A, Sarica K, Seitz C, Skolarikos A, Straub M, et al. EAU guidelines on urolithiasis. European Urology. 2021;**79**(3):464-472. DOI: 10.1016/j.eururo.2020.08.020

[32] Hall PM. Nephrolithiasis: Treatment, causes, and prevention. Cleveland Clinic Journal of Medicine. 2009;**76**(10):583-591. DOI: 10.3949/ccjm.76a.09043

[33] McAninch JW, Lue TF, editors. Smith and Tanagho's General Urology. 18th ed. New York: McGraw Hill; 2020

[34] Whitbourne K. In: Begum J, editor. Kidney Stone Surgery: Types, Risks, and Recovery. Web MD; 2024. Available from: https://www.webmd.com/kidney-stones/surgery-for-kidney-stone

[35] Wehling M, editor. Principles of Translational Science in Medicine: From Bench to Bedside. 3rd ed. Cambridge, MA: Academic Press; 2021

[36] Hamburg MA, Collins FS. The path to personalized medicine. New England Journal of Medicine. 2010;**381**(4):301-304. DOI: 10.1056/NEJMp1006304

[37] Klein JB, Nguyen CT, Saffore L, Modlin C 3rd, Modlin CS Jr. Racial disparities in urologic health care. Journal of the National Medical Association. 2008;**100**(5):508-512. DOI: 10.1016/S0027-9684(15)30498-3

[38] Fink HA, Wilt TJ, Eidman KE, Garimella PS, MacDonald R, Rutks IR, et al. Medical management to prevent recurrent nephrolithiasis in adults: A systematic review for an American

College of Physicians clinical guideline. Annals of Internal Medicine. 2013;**158**(7):535-543. DOI: 10.7326/0003-4819-158-7-201304020-00005

[39] Howles SA, Thakker RV. Genetics of kidney stone disease. Nature Reviews. Urology. 2020;**17**:407-421. DOI: 10.1038/s41585-020-0332-x

[40] Devarajan P, Murray P. Biomarkers in acute kidney injury: Are we ready for prime time? Nephron. Clinical Practice. 2014;**127**(1-4):176-179. DOI: DOIi: 10.1159/000363206

[41] Hinojosa-Gonzalez DE, Eisner BH. Biomarkers in urolithiasis. Urologic Clinics of North America. 2023;**50**(1):19-29. DOI: 10.1016/j.ucl.2022.09.004

[42] Coe FL, Evan A, Worcester E. Kidney stone disease. The Journal of Clinical Investigation. 2005;**115**(10):2598-2608. DOI: 10.1172/JCI26662

[43] Zhang F, Li W. The complex relationship between vitamin D and kidney stones: Balance, risks, and prevention strategies. Frontiers in Nutrition. 2024;**11**:1435403. DOI: 10.3389/fnut.2024.1435403

[44] Monico CG, Milliner DS. Genetic determinants of urolithiasis. Nature Reviews Nephrology. 2012;**8**(3):151-162. DOI: 10.1038/nrneph.2011.213

[45] Khan S. Role of renal epithelial cells in the initiation of calcium oxalate stones. Nephron Experimental Nephrology. 2004;**98**(2):e55-e60. DOI: 10.1159/000080257

[46] Liang D, Liu C, Yang M. The association between C-reactive protein levels and the risk of kidney stones: A population-based study. BMC Nephrology. 2024;**25**:39. DOI: 10.1186/s12882-024-03476-3

[47] Aggarwal KP, Narula S, Kakkar M, Tandon C. Nephrolithiasis: Molecular mechanism of renal stone formation and the critical role played by modulators. BioMed Research International. 2013;**2013**:292953. DOI: 10.1155/2013/292953. Epub 2013 Sep 14

[48] Worcester EM, Coe FL. Clinical practice. Calcium kidney stones. The New England Journal of Medicine. 2010;**363**(10):954-963. DOI: 10.1056/NEJMcp1001011

[49] Feng C, Liu F. Artificial intelligence in renal pathology: Current status and future. Biomolecules and Biomedicine. 2023;**23**(2):225-234. DOI: 10.17305/bjbms.2022.8318

[50] Isha S, Shah SZ. Use of artificial intelligence for analyzing kidney stone composition: Are we there yet? Mayo Clinic Proceedings: Digital Health. 2023;**1**(3):352-356. DOI: 10.1016/j.mcpdig.2023.06.007

[51] Deol ES, Kavoussi NL. Artificial intelligence applications in kidney stone disease. In: Khan SR, Gambaro G, Khan A, editors. Kidney Stone Disease. 1st ed. Amsterdam: Elsevier; 2023. pp. 169-191. DOI: 10.1016/B978-0-443-22132-3.00011-3

[52] Schönthaler M, Miernik A. Bildgebung bei urolithiasis [Imaging for urolithiasis]. Urologie. 2023;**62**(11):1144-1152. DOI: 10.1007/s00120-023-02193-3. German. Epub 2023 Sep 13

[53] Shah M, Naik N, Somani BK, Hameed BMZ. Artificial intelligence (AI) in urology—Current use and future directions: An iTRUE study. Turkish Journal of Urology. 2020;**46**(Suppl. 1): S27-S39. DOI: 10.5152/tud.2020.20117

[54] Abida R, Hussein AA, Guru KA. Artificial intelligence in urology: Current status and future perspectives. The Urologic Clinics of North America. 2024;**51**(1):117-130. DOI: 10.1016/j.ucl.2023.06.005

[55] Balawendr K, Luszezki E, Mazur A, Wyszyriska J. The multidisciplinary approach in the management of patients with kidney stone disease-a state of the art review. Nutrients. 2020;**16**(2):1932. DOI: 10.3390/nu16121932

[56] Akram M, Jahrreiss U, Skolarikos A, Geraghty R, Tzelves L, Emilliani E, et al. Urology guideline for kidney stones: Overview and comprehensive update. Journal of Clinical Medicine. 2024;**13**(4):1114. DOI: 10.3390/jcm13041114

[57] Sorensen MD, Hsi RS, Chi T, Shara N, Wactawski-Wende J, Kahn AJ, et al. Dietary intake of fiber, fruit and vegetables decreases the risk of incident kidney stones in women: A women's health initiative report. Journal of Urology. 2014;**192**:1694-1699. DOI: 10.1016/j.juro.2014.05.086

[58] Ferraro PM, Curhan GC, Taylor EN. The role of calcium in kidney stone disease: Revisiting dietary recommendations. Kidney International Reports. 2023;**8**(3):300-308. DOI: 10.1016/j.juro.2013.03.074

[59] Taylor EN, Curhan GC. Dietary factors and the risk of incident kidney stones in men: New insights after 14 years of follow-up. Journal of the American Society of Nephrology. 2008;**19**(5):853-860. DOI: 10.1097/01.ASN.0000146012.44570.20

[60] Borghi L, Meschi T, Nouvenne A, Ticinesi A. Dietary therapy in nephrolithiasis. Frontiers in Nutrition. 2021;**8**:679142. DOI: 10.3389/fnut.2021.679142

[61] Moe OW, Pearle MS, Sakhaee K. Pharmacological treatments for kidney stones: Current and emerging options. Nature Reviews Urology. 2020;**17**(7):403-419. DOI: 10.1038/nrdp.2016.8

[62] Taguchi K, Hamamoto S, Okada A. Advances in pharmacological therapies for uric acid kidney stones. Therapeutic Advances in Urology. 2023;**15**:17562872231113295. DOI: 10.1177/17562872231113295

[63] Koo K, Matlaga BR. New imaging techniques in the management of stone disease. The Urologic Clinics of North America. 2019;**46**(2):257-263. DOI: 10.1016/j.ucl.2018.12.007. Epub 2019 Mar 4

[64] Pozdzik A, Grillo V, Sakhaee K. Gaps in kidney stone disease management: From clinical theory to patient reality. Urolithiasis. 2024;**52**:61. DOI: 10.1007/s00240-024-01563-6

[65] Ticinesi A, Nouvenne A, Meschi T. Gut microbiome and kidney stone disease: Not just an oxalobacter story. Kidney International. 2019;**96**(1):25-27. DOI: 10.1016/j.kint.2019.03.020

[66] Shahmoradi L, Azizpour A, Bejani M, et al. A smartphone-based self-care application for patients with urinary tract stones: Identification of information content and functional capabilities. BMC Urology. 2022;**22**:181. DOI: 10.1186/s12894-022-01127-z

[67] Wani M, Mohamed AHA, Gareth B, Sanjeev M. Challenges and options for management of stones in anomalous kidneys: A review of current literature. Therapeutic Advances in Urology. 2023;**15**. DOI: 10.1177/17562872231217797

www.ingramcontent.com/pod-product-compliance
Lightning Source LLC
Chambersburg PA
CBHW081335190326
41458CB00018B/6005